Perspectives in Nursing 1989–1991

Perspectives in Nursing 1989–1991

National League for Nursing • New York
Pub. No. 41-2281

ISBN 0-88737-443-3

This book was set in Aster by Pageworks, Ltd. The editor and designer was Andrea Arvonio. Clarkwood Corporation was the printer and binder.

The cover was designed by Lillian Welsh.

Printed in the United States of America

CONTENTS

Nursing Centers 53

Nursing in an Urban Environment 105

Nursing Homes 133

Testing and Accreditation   *153*

Educational Mobility   *183*

PREFACE

The National League for Nursing's biennial conventions are known for the wealth of talent and expertise brought together to expand current knowledge on health care issues. The 1989 convention, held in Seattle and exploring the theme "Thriving in the '90s through Quality and Creativity," was no exception. This latest volume in the *PERSPECTIVES IN NURSING* series is published to document outstanding presentations from that convention.

The papers included here are selected "highlights" of the convention. Emphasizing innovations in education and practice designed to improve quality in nursing care and strengthen the influence of nursing on health care delivery and policy, the authors also demonstrate that nursing functions today as *the* profession of caring.

The chapters in this collection have been organized into seven sections focused preeminently on issues of quality and creativity in a variety of nursing environments. The first section, "Nursing Personnel," features research and profiles of the various nursing populations which make up NLN's constituency. The second section, "Nursing Centers," covers delivery of quality health care in these innovative settings. Further developing this theme, the authors of sections 3 and 4 discuss the special problems and rewards of "Nursing in an Urban Environment" and "Nursing Homes," specifically teaching nursing home programs. Areas in which NLN is an acknowledged leader, "Testing and Accreditation," are explored in Chapters 14 to 17; Chapters 18 to 20 describe exciting new programs for "Educational Mobility." The authors of the last and perhaps most inspiring section, "Themes and Images for the Future," offer strategies for nursing in the year 2000 and beyond planet Earth.

The issues raised, the controversies argued, and the strategies proposed for change make this volume a valuable resource for educators, researchers, practitioners, executives—all nurses, in fact, whose goal is the best possible health care system we can mutually devise. It is our hope that this volume will contribute wisdom to the continuing debate.

Sally J. Barhydt
Division of Communications
National League for Nursing

Nursing Personnel

PROFILE OF HOSPITAL NURSING PERSONNEL'S CONTEMPORARY NURSING POPULATION: FINDINGS FROM THE AMERICAN HOSPITAL ASSOCIATION'S DATA

Constance Adams, DrPH, RN
Research Program Director
American Hospital Association
Center for Nursing
Chicago, Illinois

During the 1980s, many issues evolved that impacted on the employment of nurses. The purpose of this report is to review several trends relevant to hospital-employed nursing personnel, with an emphasis on data obtained during 1987 and 1988.

Data used in this report are from surveys conducted by the American Hospital Association (AHA). Surveys of hospitals were conducted annually during the 1980s. All hospitals located in the United States were sent questionnaires for each survey and response rates were consistently just over 90%. In order to publish relevant national data, estimates were made for nonreporting hospitals and for reporting hospitals that submitted incomplete information on returned questionnaires. These estimates were based either on prior data for individual hospitals available to the AHA or on new data reported by hospitals that were similar in size, type of control, major service provided, average length of patient stay, geographic location, and other demographic characteristics.

Surveys specific to hospital-employed nursing personnel were conducted annually from 1983 through 1988. Twenty percent of all community hospitals located in the continental United States were sampled for the surveys conducted prior to December 1986 and for the one conducted in April 1987. In December 1986, 1987, and 1988, one-third of all hospitals located in the nation, including federal government hospitals, were sampled. Twenty percent of these hospitals were also sampled for the April 1988 survey. Except for the December 1986 survey, response rates for each survey declined successively from 75% in March 1983 to 52% in December 1988. The response rate to the December 1986 survey was 44%. Data from these surveys are reported only for hospitals that submitted valid information.

NUMBERS OF NURSING PERSONNEL

Numbers of all hospital-employed registered nurses increased by almost 9% between 1983 and 1987 (see Table 1) (AHA, 1984; AHA 1988). During this time, however, total numbers of hospital-employed nursing personnel remained essentially unchanged. Numbers of full-time registered nurses increased more than numbers of part-time registered nurses. Numbers of part-time licensed practical or vocational nurses increased most dramatically: The increase from 31,656 in 1983 to 65,946 in 1987 represents an overall increase of 108.3%. Numbers of full-time licensed practical or vocational nurses and numbers of all hospital-employed ancillary nursing personnel decreased between 1983 and 1987.

FULL-TIME EQUIVALENT (FTE) POSITIONS

Budgeted Positions

According to hospital nursing personnel survey data (Adams, 1989), budgeted full-time equivalent (FTE) positions for hospital-employed registered nurses increased more than budgeted FTE positions for other categories of nursing personnel during calendar year 1987 (see Table 2). The mean increase in registered nurse budgeted positions was 4.7; for licensed practical nurses it was 0.3 and for nurse aides or orderlies it was 1.0. On the one hand, slightly more than 45% of the hospitals responding to the 1988 survey increased their numbers of budgeted FTE positions for registered nurses; on the other, nurse aide or orderly budgeted FTE positions were eliminated during the same time by more hospitals than other types of nursing personnel positions.

Greatest increases in budgeted FTE positions for registered nurses during 1987 took place in hospitals located in small urban areas, nonprofit hospitals, and hospitals with 500 or more inpatient beds (see Table 3) (Adams, 1989). Greatest increases in budgeted FTE positions for all categories of hospital-employed nursing personnel took place in hospitals located in the East South Central region of the United States. Budgeted FTE positions for licensed practical nurses and nurse aides or orderlies also increased the most in hospitals with 300 to 399 beds. Such positions for nurse aides or orderlies also increased the most in investor-owned hospitals.

Filled Positions

Between 1983 and 1987, the number of filled positions for hospital-employed registered nurses increased by 9% while the number of filled positions for all nursing personnel decreased by 2% (see Table 4) (AHA, 1988). Percentages of filled FTE positions for registered nurses increased most dramatically between 1985 and 1987 in hospitals with 500 or more inpatient beds and in hospitals located in the East South Central region of the country (see Table 5) (AHA, 1986; AHA, 1988). Percentages of filled FTE positions for licensed practical or vocational nurses decreased most during this period in metropolitan hospitals, hospitals with 100 to 199 inpatient beds, and hospitals located in the East North Central region. Percentages of filled FTE positions for ancillary nursing personnel decreased most in nonmetropolitan hospitals, hospitals with 500 or more inpatient beds, and hospitals located in the East South Central region.

NURSING PERSONNEL SHORTAGES

Degree of Shortages

Percentages of those hospitals surveyed that reported "severe" shortages of staff registered nurses decreased between April 1987 and April 1988 (see Table 6) (Adams, 1989; Center for Nursing, 1987; Minnock & Young, 1987). Instead, more hospitals reported overall shortages to be "moderate" or "mild." Almost 24% of these hospitals reported "no" shortages in April 1987 compared with 21% in April 1988. In April 1988, registered nurse staff shortages were considered to be "moderate" by about 51% of the hospitals that reported shortages of staff registered nurses (see Table 7) (Adams, 1989). "Severe" shortages were most prevalent in rural hospitals, hospitals located in the West South Central region of the United States, federal government hospitals, and hospitals with less than 50 inpatient beds.

Vacancy rates for hospital-budgeted registered nurse staff positions fluctuated between 1984 and 1988 (see Figure 1) (Adams, 1989). Rates derived from hospital nursing personnel surveys conducted in December 1986, 1987, and 1988 were consistently higher than rates derived from comparable surveys conducted at other times of the year. In April 1988, the vacancy rate in responding hospitals for registered nurses was 7.6%; for licensed practical nurses, 2.8%; and for nurse aides or orderlies, 3.0% (see Table 8) (Adams, 1989). In December 1988, the vacancy rate for registered nurses in responding hospitals was 10.6% (see Table 9) (Adams, 1989).

Registered nurse vacancy rates for hospitals that responded to the April and December 1988 hospital nursing personnel surveys were highest in nonfederal government hospitals and in hospitals with less that 50 inpatient beds. Regions of the country with the highest registered nurse vacancy rates during both time periods were the Mid-Atlantic, East North Central, and Pacific regions. The region with the highest registered nurse vacancy rate among December survey

FIGURE 1

Hospital-Employed RN Vacancy Rates for Specified Years and Months

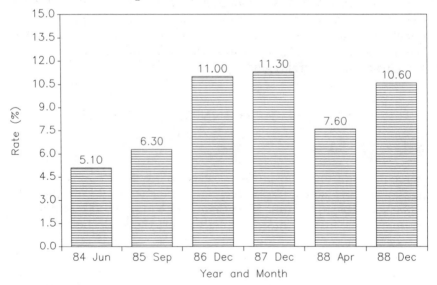

SOURCE: Adams, C. (1989). *Hospital nursing personnel, 1988.* Chicago: American Hospital Association.

reporting hospitals was the West South Central region; however, the same rate for this region among April reporting hospitals was much lower.

Vacancy rates for licensed practical nurses and nurse aides or orderlies in April 1988 survey responding hospitals were highest for hospitals located in small urban areas and in hospitals located in New England. Licensed practical nurse vacancy rates were also highest in government hospitals and in hospitals with less than 50 inpatient beds or 500 or more inpatient beds. Nurse aide or orderly vacancy rates were highest in nonprofit hospitals and hospitals with 400 or more inpatient beds.

Turnovers

In April 1988, among respondents to the hospital nursing personnel survey, the turnover rate for registered nurses was 18.7%; for licensed practical nurses, 15.0%; and for nurse aides or orderlies, 17.9% (see Table 10) (Adams, 1989). Within these hospitals, essentially one in five registered nurses terminated employment in a given institution during 1987. Fewer licensed practical or vocational nurses and nurse aides or orderlies terminated employment.

Turnover rates for all categories of hospital-employed nursing personnel were highest in hospitals located in large urban areas. Registered nurse turnover rates were highest in hospitals located in the West South Central and Pacific regions of the United States, as well as in investor-owned hospitals. Turnover rates for licensed practical nurses were highest in hospitals located in the Mountain region, federal hospitals, and hospitals with 100 to 199 inpatient beds. Comparable rates for nurse aides or orderlies were highest for hospitals located in the Mountain region, investor-owned hospitals, and hospitals with 100 to 199 inpatient beds.

Differences Between Newly Hired and Terminated Personnel

Although turnover rates seem high, especially for registered nurses, mean differences between newly hired and terminated personnel during 1987 were positive for all categories of nursing personnel (see Tables 11 and 12) (Adams, 1989). Most hospitals responding to the April 1988 hospital nursing personnel survey employed larger numbers of nursing personnel, particularly registered nurses, at the end of 1987 than they did at the beginning of 1987. Numbers of licensed practical nurses decreased in some hospitals more frequently than numbers of other categories of nursing personnel. Numbers of full-time registered nurses increased most dramatically during 1987 in hospitals located in large urban areas, New England or the Mid-Atlantic region of the United States, nonprofit hospitals, and hospitals with 400 or more inpatient beds. Except for the addition of part-time nurse aides or orderlies in some hospitals with 500 or more inpatient beds, mean differences between newly hired and terminated licensed practical nurses and nurse aides or orderlies were negligible.

Length of Employment for Full-Time Registered Nurses

Historically, large numbers of full-time registered nurses employed by respondents to the hospital nursing personnel survey have been employed for 5 or more years and this trend appears to be continuing (see Figure 2) (Adams, 1989). Between 1984 and 1988, there was a slight increase in the percentage of those employed for less than 1 year and slight decreases in the percentages of those employed for at least 1 year but less than 5 years.

FIGURE **2**
**Full-Time RN Employment for Specified
Years, by Length of Employment**

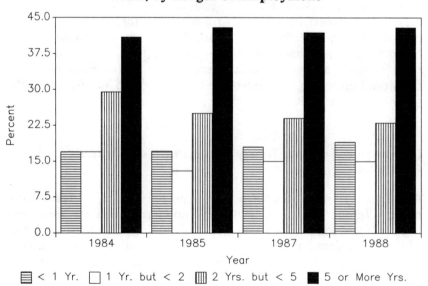

source: Adams, C. (1989). *Hospital nursing personnel, 1988*. Chicago: American Hospital Association.

Almost 69% of the full-time registered nurses employed by hospitals that responded to the April 1988 survey had been employed for 2 or more years (see Table 13) (Adams, 1989). Part-time registered nurses had been employed for fewer years than full-time hospital-employed registered nurses.

Length of Time Required to Recruit Nursing Personnel

Registered nurse positions that required more than 90 days to fill by at least 30% of all hospitals responding to the April 1988 hospital nursing personnel survey were clinical specialist, medical surgical staff, head nurse, labor and delivery staff, and nursing supervisor or assistant administrator positions (see Table 14) (Adams, 1989). Positions requiring the least amount of time to fill were home health staff positions, emergency room staff positions, and psychiatric staff positions. Budgeted positions that did not require filling most frequently were clinical specialist and home health staff positions.

SUMMARY

Numbers of hospital-employed registered nurses and the number of filled FTE positions for registered nurses increased by about 9% between 1983 and 1987. During this same period of time, total numbers of hospital-employed nursing personnel remained essentially unchanged and the number of filled FTE positions for these personnel decreased by 2%. The mean increase in budgeted FTE positions for registered nurses during calendar year 1987 was 4.7, while mean increases in budgeted FTE positions for practical nurses and nurse aides or orderlies were much smaller.

Percentages of hospitals reporting "severe" shortages of staff registered nurses decreased between April 1987 and April 1988. By April 1988, registered nurse staff shortages were considered to be "moderate" by about 51% of respondents that reported having shortages.

The registered nurse vacancy rate in survey responding hospitals was 7.6% in April 1988 and 10.6% in December 1988. Between 1984 and 1988, vacancy rates derived from surveys conducted in December 1986, 1987, and 1988 were consistently higher (10.6–11.3%) than rates derived from comparable surveys conducted at other times of the year (5.1–7.6%). Registered nurse vacancy rates were highest in 1988 for nonfederal government hospitals and in hospitals with less than 50 inpatient beds.

In April 1988, the turnover rate in survey responding hospitals for registered nurses was 18.7% meaning that essentially one in five of these nurses terminated employment within a given institution during the previous year. At the same time, almost 69% of all full-time registered nurses employed by these hospitals had been employed for at least 2 years and 46.2% had been employed for 5 or more years. Mean differences between newly hired and terminated personnel during 1987 were positive for all categories of nursing personnel. Most responding hospitals had larger numbers of nursing personnel, particularly registered nurses, at the end of 1987 than they did at the beginning of that year.

Registered nurse positions that were the most difficult to fill were head nurse positions and medical surgical staff positions. Those that required filling least often were clinical specialist and home health staff positions.

REFERENCES

Adams, C. (1989). *Hospital nursing personnel, 1988.* Chicago: American Hospital Association.

American Hospital Association. (1984). *Hospital statistics.* Chicago: Author.

American Hospital Association. (1986). *Hospital statistics.* Chicago: Author.

American Hospital Association. (1988). *Hospital statistics.* Chicago: Author.

Center for Nursing. (1987). *Report of the 1987 hospital nursing demand survey.* Chicago: American Hospital Association.

Minnock, A., & Young, W. B. (1987). *Report of hospital nursing personnel survey 1987.* Chicago: American Hospital Association.

TABLE 1

Hospital-Employed Nursing Personnel, by Personnel Type and Full-Time or Part-Time Work Status, 1983 and 1987

	1983		1987		
Personnel Type	No.	%	No.	%	Percent Change
Registered nurses					
Full-time	623,693	68.6	682,955	69.1	+9.5
Part-time	285,706	31.4	305,874	30.9	+7.1
Total	909,399	100.0	988,829	100.0	+8.7
Licensed practical or vocational nurses					
Full-time	215,881	87.2	168,284	71.8	−22.0
Part-time	31,656	12.8	65,946	28.2	+108.3
Total	247,537	100.0	234,230	100.0	−5.4
Ancillary nursing personnel					
Full-time	351,446	77.9	292,327	77.4	−16.8
Part-time	99,678	22.1	85,530	22.6	−14.2
Total	451,124	100.0	377,857	100.0	−16.2
All nursing personnel					
Full-time	1,191,020	74.1	1,143,566	71.4	−4.0
Part-time	417,040	25.9	457,350	28.6	+9.7
Total	1,608,060	100.0	1,600,916	100.0	−0.4

Sources: American Hospital Association. (1984). *Hospital statistics*. Chicago: Author. American Hospital Association. (1988). *Hospital statistics*. Chicago: Author.

TABLE 2

Changes in Budgeted Full-Time Equivalent (FTE) Positions for Hospital-Employed Nursing Personnel During 1987, by Personnel Type

		Percent of Hospitals			
Personnel Type	No. of Hosp.	Decrease	No Change	Increase	Mean Change in FTEs
Registered nurses	742	10.8	43.9	45.3	+4.7
Licensed practical nurses	712	17.2	57.3	25.0	+0.3
Nurse aides or orderlies	710	19.4	52.1	28.5	+1.0

Source: Adams, C. (1989). *Hospital nursing personnel, 1988*. Chicago: American Hospital Association.

TABLE 3

Mean Changes in Budgeted Full-Time Equivalent (FTE) Positions for Hospital-Employed Nursing Personnel During 1987, by Personnel Type and Hospital Characteristics

Hospital Characteristics	Registered Nurses		Licensed Practical Nurses		Nurse Aides or Orderlies	
	No. of Hosp.	Mean Change	No. of Hosp.	Mean Change	No. of Hosp.	Mean Change
Location						
Rural	304	+1.5	294	+0.1	293	+0.4
Urban (<1,000,000)	238	+8.8	230	+0.8	232	+1.4
Urban (≥1,000,000)	200	+4.8	188	+0.1	185	+1.5
Region						
New England	39	+5.3	37	+1.6	40	+1.2
Mid-Atlantic	90	+6.3	88	+0.6	87	+2.4
South Atlantic	102	+6.8	99	−0.2	100	+1.4
East North Central	127	+6.8	121	+0.4	119	+0.1
East South Central	48	+8.4	46	+2.5	47	+2.7
West North Central	104	+5.8	99	+0.2	101	+0.5
West South Central	90	+2.9	90	−0.3	87	+0.2
Mountain	56	+4.9	52	−0.2	50	+0.5
Pacific	86	+2.6	80	+0.2	79	+1.1
Type of organization						
Government (federal)	44	+1.0	41	+0.1	40	+0.1
Government (nonfederal)	208	+3.0	204	+0.3	204	−0.6
Investor-owned	77	+4.0	74	+1.5	73	+3.6
Nonprofit	413	+6.2	393	+0.1	393	+1.2
Number of inpatient beds						
1–49	148	+0.9	139	0.0	134	+0.4
50–99	165	+1.1	160	+0.4	164	+0.5
100–199	148	+2.4	141	+0.2	140	+0.7
200–299	99	+5.6	98	+0.7	98	+1.3
300–399	69	+13.4	64	+1.4	65	+3.9
400–499	43	+4.2	41	−0.9	41	+1.7
500+	70	+16.3	69	+0.3	68	+0.6
Total	742	+4.7	712	+0.3	710	+1.0

SOURCE: Adams, C. (1989). *Hospital nursing personnel, 1988.* Chicago: American Hospital Association.

TABLE **4**

Filled Full-Time Equivalent (FTE) Hospital-Employed Nursing Personnel Positions, by Personnel Type, 1983 and 1987

Personnel Type	Filled FTE Positions		
	1983	1987	Change, %
Registered nurses	766,546	835,892	+9.0
Licensed practical or vocational nurses	231,709	201,257	−13.1
Ancillary nursing personnel	401,285	335,092	−16.5
All nursing personnel	1,399,540	1,372,241	−2.0

SOURCE: American Hospital Association. (1988). *Hospital statistics.* Chicago: Author.

TABLE **5**

Percentages of Filled Full-Time Equivalent (FTE) Hospital-Employed Nursing Personnel Positions, by Personnel Type and Hospital Characteristics, 1985 and 1987

Hospital Character-istics	Personnel Type								
	Registered Nurses, %			Licensed Practical or Vocational Nurses, %			Ancillary Nursing Personnel, %		
	1985	1987	Diff	1985	1987	Diff	1985	1987	Diff
Location									
Metropolitan	52.2	54.7	+2.5	24.4	23.2	−1.2	23.4	22.1	−1.3
Non-metropolitan	64.7	67.2	+2.5	14.9	12.9	−2.0	20.4	19.8	−0.6
Region									
New England	61.1	63.0	+1.9	14.0	12.4	−1.6	24.9	24.6	−0.3
Mid-Atlantic	59.0	60.7	−1.7	13.4	12.4	−1.0	27.6	26.9	−0.7
South Atlantic	56.2	59.4	+3.2	16.7	15.4	−1.3	27.1	25.2	−1.9
East North Central	60.8	63.6	+2.8	14.6	12.6	−2.0	24.5	23.8	−0.7
East South Central	50.7	55.0	+4.3	20.8	19.1	−1.7	28.5	25.9	−2.6
West North Central	59.3	62.7	+3.4	15.8	14.0	−1.8	24.8	23.3	−1.5
West South Central	50.3	52.5	+2.2	22.6	21.5	−1.1	27.1	26.0	−1.1

Mountain	64.3	66.4	+2.1	14.4	12.8	−1.6	21.3	20.9	−0.4
Pacific	63.9	66.1	+2.2	15.6	13.7	−1.9	20.5	20.2	−0.3

Number of inpatient beds

1–49	46.8	49.2	+2.4	21.1	20.9	−0.2	32.0	29.8	−2.2
50–99	52.1	54.6	+2.5	21.8	20.8	−1.0	26.1	24.6	−1.5
100–199	57.0	59.7	+2.7	19.7	17.6	−2.1	23.2	22.7	−0.5
200–299	61.4	63.1	+1.7	16.9	15.2	−1.7	21.7	21.7	0.0
300–399	64.0	65.6	+1.6	15.1	13.3	−1.8	21.0	21.1	+0.1
400–499	62.3	63.8	+1.5	13.7	12.1	−1.6	23.9	24.0	+0.1
500+	55.7	59.8	+3.1	13.3	11.9	−1.4	30.9	28.3	−2.6
Total	58.3	60.9	+2.6	16.2	14.7	−1.5	25.5	24.4	−1.1

SOURCES: American Hospital Association. (1986). *Hospital statistics.* Chicago: Author.
American Hospital Association. (1988). *Hospital statistics.* Chicago: Author.

TABLE **6**
Degree of Hospital Staff Registered Nurse Shortages, by Applicable Month, 1987 and 1988

Month and Year	No. of Hosp.	Degree of Staff Registered Nurse Shortages, %			
		None	Mild	Moderate	Severe
April 1987	719	23.8	21.9	35.5	18.8
December 1987	1,447	21.4	25.7	39.1	13.8
April 1988	796	21.0	26.9	40.3	11.8

SOURCES: Adams, C. (1989). *Hospital Nursing Personnel, 1988.* Chicago: American Hospital Association.
Center for Nursing. (1987). *Report of the 1987 hospital nursing demand survey.* Chicago: American Hospital Association.
Minnock, A. & Young, W. B. (1987). *Report of hospital nursing personnel survey 1987.* Chicago: American Hospital Association.

TABLE 7
Degree of Hospital-Employed Staff Registered Nurse Shortages, by Hospital Characteristics, April 1988

Hospital Characteristics	No. of Hosp.		% Yes	Shortage Severity for for Hospitals Reporting Shortages, %		
	No	Yes	Yes	Mild	Mod	Severe
Location						
Rural	82	245	74.9	33.6	50.0	16.4
Urban (<1,000,000)	49	205	80.7	40.6	43.0	16.4
Urban (≥1,000,000)	36	179	83.3	27.2	55.6	17.2
Region						
New England	6	39	86.7	53.7	29.3	17.1
Mid-Atlantic	11	83	88.3	31.0	51.2	17.9
South Atlantic	22	93	80.9	23.7	59.1	17.2
East North Central	31	101	76.5	33.3	52.9	13.7
East South Central	8	41	83.7	37.5	45.0	17.5
West North Central	39	72	64.9	40.8	43.4	15.8
West South Central	19	77	80.2	27.3	49.4	23.4
Mountain	14	44	75.9	28.3	58.7	13.0
Pacific	17	79	82.3	42.3	43.6	14.1
Type of organization						
Government (federal)	12	34	73.9	30.3	57.6	12.1
Government (nonfederal)	58	167	74.2	31.8	47.1	21.2
Investor-owned	15	67	81.7	32.8	55.2	11.9
Nonprofit	82	361	81.5	35.7	48.5	15.8
Number of inpatient beds						
1–49	46	113	71.1	33.3	45.6	21.1
50–99	43	135	75.8	39.9	46.4	13.8
100–199	29	128	81.5	34.9	51.2	14.0
200–299	19	93	82.1	30.1	59.1	10.8
300–399	15	59	79.7	29.5	55.7	14.8
400–499	9	36	80.0	40.5	29.7	29.7
500+	6	65	91.5	27.7	49.2	23.1
Total	167	629	79.0	34.1	50.9	15.0

Source: Adams, C. (1989). *Hospital nursing personnel, 1988.* Chicago: American Hospital Association.

TABLE 8

Full-Time Equivalent (FTE) Vacancy Rates for Hospital-Employed Nursing Personnel, by Personnel Type and Hospital Characteristics, April 1988

Hospital Characteristics	Registered Nurses		Licensed Practical Nurses		Nurse Aides or Orderlies	
	No. of Hosp.	Rate	No. of Hosp.	Rate	No. of Hosp.	Rate
Location						
Rural	234	9.5	211	3.0	208	1.1
Urban (<1,000,000)	163	6.6	149	3.1	148	3.6
Urban (≥1,000,000)	124	8.0	115	2.7	109	3.1
Region						
New England	21	8.1	21	11.3	21	11.3
Mid-Atlantic	62	11.1	56	5.8	55	4.0
South Atlantic	62	10.8	54	3.8	52	2.5
East North Central	88	5.7	79	1.9	77	1.9
East South Central	34	11.3	34	3.2	35	3.9
West North Central	90	4.0	77	1.5	77	2.3
West South Central	66	5.9	62	0.5	56	0.7
Mountain	40	4.7	37	2.3	39	1.6
Pacific	58	11.3	55	6.0	53	9.3
Type of organization						
Government (federal)	24	5.8	22	6.0	22	2.7
Government (nonfederal)	163	10.0	149	6.0	147	3.0
Investor-owned	53	6.2	46	0.5	45	0.7
Nonprofit	281	7.3	258	2.4	251	3.9
Number of inpatient beds						
1–49	125	10.1	115	4.7	114	1.8
50–99	128	6.9	116	3.5	114	3.9
100–199	104	5.3	91	1.3	91	2.2
200–299	65	8.5	62	3.6	60	3.6
300–399	41	6.5	37	2.2	35	1.8
400–499	22	11.1	18	1.9	17	5.8
500+	36	8.7	36	5.4	34	4.1
Total	521	7.6	475	2.8	465	3.0

SOURCE: Adams, C. (1989). *Hospital nursing personnel, 1988*. Chicago: American Hospital Association.

TABLE 9
Full-Time Equivalent (FTE) Vacancy Rates for Hospital-Employed Registered Nurses, by Hospital Characteristics, December 1988

Hospital Characteristics	No. of Hosp.	Registered Nurses, Rate
Location		
Rural	542	10.3
Urban (<1,000,000)	361	10.3
Urban (≥1,000,000)	299	11.1
Region		
New England	77	8.5
Mid-Atlantic	126	10.2
South Atlantic	194	12.3
East North Central	201	7.2
East South Central	96	11.0
West North Central	165	6.9
West South Central	149	16.7
Mountain	64	9.6
Pacific	130	12.4
Type of organization		
Government (federal)	70	12.5
Government (nonfederal)	353	15.2
Investor-owned	119	10.0
Nonprofit	660	9.0
Number of inpatient beds		
1–49	244	14.3
50–99	289	10.3
100–199	275	10.5
200–299	151	8.1
300–399	89	12.8
400–499	53	11.7
500+	101	10.4
Total	1,202	10.6

SOURCE: Adams, C. (1989). *Hospital nursing personnel, 1988.* Chicago: American Hospital Association.

TABLE 10

Full-Time Equivalent (FTE) Turnover Rates for Hospital-Employed Nursing Personnel, by Personnel Type and Hospital Characteristics, April 1988

Hospital Characteristics	Registered Nurses		Licensed Practical Nurses		Nurse Aides or Orderlies	
	No. of Hosp.	Rate	No. of Hosp.	Rate	No. of Hosp.	Rate
Location						
Rural	193	17.5	176	15.1	169	15.0
Urban (<1,000,000)	97	18.4	94	14.2	89	19.1
Urban (≥1,000,000)	78	19.6	68	16.2	63	18.5
Region						
New England	12	16.3	13	10.4	11	22.0
Mid-Atlantic	48	18.4	44	14.2	41	15.2
South Atlantic	41	21.5	35	18.5	34	17.9
East North Central	63	14.7	58	12.4	54	14.2
East South Central	24	20.9	22	16.3	20	21.4
West North Central	62	14.0	55	11.3	56	22.4
West South Central	51	22.0	49	15.9	46	20.2
Mountain	30	22.1	29	26.7	30	30.0
Pacific	37	21.4	33	15.1	29	17.6
Type of organization						
Government (federal)	19	19.6	17	20.0	14	13.5
Government (nonfederal)	120	19.3	108	15.9	105	14.8
Investor-owned	32	24.9	28	15.3	28	30.8
Nonprofit	197	18.0	185	13.6	174	20.2
Number of inpatient beds						
1–49	97	21.5	90	13.7	84	17.8
50–99	99	14.0	92	15.0	91	15.6
100–199	62	21.5	53	17.4	55	23.6
200–299	43	20.4	41	13.7	35	20.6
300–399	25	18.4	23	14.0	22	18.1
400–499	18	20.1	15	14.8	14	15.8
500+	24	17.2	24	15.7	20	16.2
Total	368	18.7	338	15.0	321	17.9

SOURCE: Adams, C. (1989). *Hospital nursing personnel, 1988.* Chicago: American Hospital Association.

TABLE 11

Differences Between Newly Hired and Terminated Full-Time Hospital-Employed Nursing Personnel during Calendar Year 1987, by Personnel Type and Hospital Characteristics, April 1988

Hospital Characteristics	Registered Nurses		Licensed Practical Nurses		Nurse Aides or Orderlies	
	No. of Hosp.	Mean Change	No. of Hosp.	Mean Change	No. of Hosp.	Mean Change
Location						
Rural	246	1.1	222	0.2	209	0.5
Urban (<1,000,000)	138	5.7	131	0.3	116	1.0
Urban (≥1,000,000)	112	9.7	96	0.4	87	2.2
Region						
New England	21	7.9	19	0.4	19	5.4
Mid-Atlantic	60	7.4	57	1.1	55	1.0
South Atlantic	65	3.8	59	−0.7	53	2.3
East North Central	79	4.9	73	0.2	68	−0.2
East South Central	33	2.9	32	−0.1	28	0.2
West North Central	79	2.0	70	0.6	66	0.9
West South Central	71	4.2	62	1.0	56	0.8
Mountain	37	3.0	34	0.2	30	0.1
Pacific	51	4.3	43	−0.5	37	0.5
Type of organization						
Government (federal)	33	0.8	32	0.3	25	0.3
Government (nonfederal)	166	2.4	153	0.1	147	1.3
Investor-owned	48	3.0	39	0.6	34	1.6
Nonprofit	249	6.3	225	0.3	206	0.7
Number of inpatient beds						
1–49	124	0.2	110	0.4	100	0.2
50–99	126	1.3	111	0.6	104	0.4
100–199	96	0.9	88	−0.5	79	0.0
200–299	59	5.2	56	0.9	52	0.8
300–399	33	9.2	32	−0.2	29	1.7
400–499	26	21.6	22	0.8	21	4.8
500+	32	21.4	30	−1.4	27	5.2
Total	496	4.3	449	0.3	412	1.0

SOURCE: Adams, C. (1989). *Hospital nursing personnel, 1988.* Chicago: American Hospital Association.

TABLE 12
Differences Between Newly Hired and Terminated Part-Time Hospital-Employed Nursing Personnel during Calendar Year 1987, by Personnel Type and Hospital Characteristics, April 1988

Hospital Characteristics	Registered Nurses		Licensed Practical Nurses		Nurse Aides or Orderlies	
	No. of Hosp.	Mean Change	No. of Hosp.	Mean Change	No. of Hosp.	Mean Change
Location						
Rural	194	0.4	189	0.6	185	1.3
Urban (<1,000,000)	103	3.4	101	0.3	100	4.0
Urban (≥1,000,000)	80	−0.4	78	−0.2	77	3.0
Region						
New England	18	1.7	18	−0.8	15	2.3
Mid-Atlantic	52	0.3	50	0.9	49	2.4
South Atlantic	43	−0.7	43	0.0	42	1.8
East North Central	63	−0.5	61	−0.1	60	1.8
East South Central	26	4.5	24	2.4	24	3.2
West North Central	64	0.1	63	0.8	63	1.5
West South Central	48	3.3	46	0.2	46	2.7
Mountain	29	1.0	29	0.2	29	0.4
Pacific	34	2.7	34	−0.4	34	6.9
Type of organization						
Government (federal)	20	0.1	19	0.0	19	1.8
Government (nonfederal)	130	1.5	125	0.4	122	2.7
Investor-owned	28	2.2	27	0.3	27	1.7
Nonprofit	199	0.6	197	0.3	194	2.4
Number of inpatient beds						
1–49	88	0.4	86	0.2	84	1.0
50–99	98	0.8	95	0.5	94	1.0
100–199	73	1.9	72	0.5	72	1.6
200–299	48	0.2	47	0.4	45	4.2
300–399	27	−0.8	26	−0.7	26	0.9
400–499	19	0.0	18	−0.4	18	−1.2
500+	24	5.7	24	0.3	23	17.2
Total	377	1.0	368	0.3	362	2.4

SOURCE: Adams, C. (1989). *Hospital nursing personnel, 1988.* Chicago: American Hospital Association.

TABLE 13
TABLE 13
Length of Employment for Hospital-Employed Registered Nurses, April 1988

Length of Employment	Full-Time		Part-Time	
	No. of Hosp.	Mean Percent	No. of Hosp.	Mean Percent
Less than 1 year	520	17.9	441	21.3
1 year or more but less than 2 years	520	13.7	439	15.0
2 years or more but less than 5 years	521	22.3	441	21.9
5 or more years	521	46.2	441	39.4

SOURCE: Adams, C. (1989). *Hospital nursing personnel, 1988*. Chicago: American Hospital Association.

TABLE 14
Length of Time Required to Recruit Registered Nurses for Specific Types of Positions, April 1988

Type of Position	No. of Hospitals	Length of Time Required by Hospitals to Recruit, %			
		1*	2	3	4
Clinical specialist	338	14.2	16.9	35.2	33.7
Emergency room staff	627	33.5	26.8	24.6	15.2
Medical surgical staff	707	25.3	33.8	36.2	4.7
Head nurse	611	16.7	26.4	48.9	8.0
Home health staff	338	44.7	14.5	9.8	31.1
Intensive care or critical care staff	714	28.0	26.9	25.6	19.5
Labor and delivery staff	507	28.4	25.0	33.9	12.6
Pediatric staff	439	28.2	25.3	28.2	18.2
Psychiatric staff	349	33.2	29.8	21.2	15.8
Operating room staff	663	30.6	24.9	28.2	16.3
Nursing supervisor or assistant administrator	683	21.7	22.4	30.3	25.6

* 1 = Less than 60 days
  2 = 60 to 90 days
  3 = More than 90 days
  4 = Did not recruit for position

SOURCE: Adams, C. (1989). *Hospital nursing personnel, 1988*. Chicago: American Hospital Association.

THE MANY FACES OF THE NEWLY LICENSED NURSE

Peri Rosenfeld, PhD
Vice President, Research
National League for Nursing
New York, New York

The last few years have presented some new and complex challenges for the nursing community. In 1984, the NLN's annual survey found that enrollments had suddenly dropped. While decreasing enrollments in diploma programs had been expected, ADN and BSN programs had had fairly healthy enrollment until this unanticipated turn of events.

The situation worsened for the next few years, and in addition to the enrollment crisis, hospitals were reporting unusually high vacancy rates. Hence, the nation was made aware of the nursing shortage. There is some good news, however. The results of the 1988 annual survey indicate that there has been an improvement in admissions to nursing educational programs (see Figure 1). The 4.5% increase in admissions is a sign in the right direction, but, certainly, there needs to be greater improvement to return us to the pre-1984 levels. Similarly, enrollments have stabilized and bounced back a bit (about 1% increase), but the current number of enrollments—almost 186,000—still represents a loss of over 60,000 nursing students since 1984 when the number of enrollments was about 250,000. The 1989 annual survey will help assess whether this upward trend will continue.

Much has been written since the nursing shortage became "big news." Journalists, economists, social scientists, government officials, and even physicians (!) have had a lot to say about nursing. More importantly, nurses have voiced their positions in blue-ribbon commissions and reports throughout the nation. In many of these discussions, there has been a preponderance of anecdotal and experiential information given; while these are valuable sources of information, they are no substitute for empirical, verifiable data.

This need for reliable data on nurses was one of the motivating factors behind conducting the newly licensed nurse project. The National League for Nursing wished to take a leadership role in providing vital data for both educators and administrators to use and understand the current cohort of new faces within the nursing profession and hence to better recruit and retain the students and RNs in their institutions. Put another way, a study of newly licensed nurses would be both an outcome measure of our nursing educational institutions as well as a guide for understanding the future nursing supply.

First, a few words about methodology. In February 1988, 53,000 surveys were sent to all those who had successfully passed NCLEX-RN in July 1987. Hence, about 7 months after entering the nursing work-force, we surveyed the newly licensed nurses as to their educational and employment experiences. After three waves of mailings and over 700 carefully selected telephone interviews, a national response rate of over 70% was achieved. In short, over 38,000 new RNs responded; item response rates were excellent. Even sensitive areas such as salary and age garnered response rates over 90%. Analysis of nonresponse found that only one area may be slightly biased—the proportion of blacks is underrepresented by 1%. Notwithstanding this limitation, the data are vastly valid and reliable.

There is a great deal of information in the newly licensed nurse report and it can be grouped into four global categories: (1) educational characteristics, (2) demographic characteristics, (3) employment experiences, and (4) geographic mobility. In addition to the empirical data, we received numerous letters from newly licensed nurses giving us some qualitative information with which to gain greater insights about their experiences. For now, I would like to offer an overview of some of the major findings and to interpret the data in the context of the changing health care and higher educational systems.

First, (Figure 2) the proportion of new RNs who have graduated from the different programs types is key—53% with associate degrees, 34% with baccalaureate degrees, and 13% with diplomas. While many of us are aware of the increasing proportion of associate degree grads among the recent cohorts of new RNs, it is less obvious that this trend alone has profound implications.

AD grads are demographically thoroughly different creatures from their BSN or diploma counterparts, and these demographic differences are strongly correlated with different educational and employment behaviors.

Marital Status. (Figure 3) Almost 60% of the ADs are married whereas almost 60% of the BSN/Diploma grads are single. Similarly over 50% of the AD grads have dependent children living at home—far smaller numbers of the other grads have obligations associated with children.

Age. The marital status data can be explained to some extent by the age differences (Figure 4). The median age for BSN/Diploma grads is 23, suggesting that most of these individuals go on to nursing school soon after high school.

The median age for AD grads is 31, suggesting that the decision to pursue a career in nursing came later in life. The age distribution is revealing. The mode or peak age for BSNs is about 23 and about 22 for diploma graduates. Among AD grads, the peak does not appear until the late 20s and early 30s. Moreover, a greater number of AD grads are in the 40+ category.

These demographic characteristics affect labor force participation in a variety of ways which will be elaborated upon later. However, before leaving this topic of variations among graduates of the different program types, I want to share a unique piece of data.

LPNs. (Figure 5) When asked if they had previously held an LPN/LVN license, a surprising 41% of the AD grads responded "yes," whereas only 12% of the diploma and 8% BSNs responded this way. Note that the question did not ask, "Have you ever *practiced* as an LPN/LVN?" However, the data are still very revealing as to the different educational paths of our new RNs.

Employment Status. (Figure 6) Over 97% of newly licensed nurses were employed in nursing positions. Of these 72% were not seeking other employment, 24% were seeking *another* nursing job, and 2.5% were seeking a non-nursing job.

In short, these data show strong and loyal laborforce participation among new nurses. Additionally, there are no significant differences among graduates of the different program types vis-à-vis employment status.

In terms of *activity status*, we found that over 90% of the BSN graduates are employed full-time whereas 79% of the AD grads are full-timers. This is a function of some of the demographic characteristics described earlier.

Despite the enormous growth in health care *settings* that employ RNs, over 90% of the new nurses have chosen hospital positions (Figure 7). This may be partially explained by (1) higher salaries are offered by hospitals, (2) many other health care settings require some hospital experience as a requirement for employment, and (3) many new RNs accept positions in those agencies in which they received their clinical preparation. We found that almost 80% found jobs before graduation.

Salaries (Figure 8) vary region by region, with the highest average salaries in the Pacific, New England, and Mid-Atlantic regions. On a state level, California and Connecticut offer the highest salaries. Nationally the average salary for a new RN (full-time) is about $22,500.

We also queried new RNs about two subjective areas: (1) job satisfaction and (2) perceptions of the adequacy of their nursing education in preparing them for their current job. We found the following:

Job satisfaction (Figure 9) Many new RNs wrote letters about the frightening working conditions in which they practice, conditions that breed resentment and anger. However, the majority (64%) stated that, in general, they were satisfied in their current job. The third that stated dissatisfaction were asked to assess the main reason for their dissatisfaction. Inadequate salary (40%) was the most frequently cited reason and working conditions (22%) was the second reason for dissatisfaction (Figure 10).

Perhaps the most distressing finding was in the area of perceived adequacy of nursing education in preparing new RNs for their current jobs. In Figure 11 note that all graduates from all program types found their classroom experiences to be adequate. However, wide differences are uncovered in the clinical experiences. Some have surmised that the lower numbers for BSN graduates are due to the fact that their clinical preparation was more diverse than the diploma or AD grad and hence hospital employment is least satisfying for the BSN grad who had been prepared to practice in the community/public health arena. Unfortunately, when we analyzed the data further, it was found that even those BSN graduates employed in alternative health care settings continued to report inadequacies in their clinical preparations.

Clearly, this is an area that requires further research to better understand what factors influence these perceptions and how actual educational experiences are interpreted in the workplace.

A detailed and comprehensive report of the findings of the Newly Licensed Nurse survey is available in the NLN publication, *Profiles of the Newly Licensed Nurse*, which was published in July 1989. In addition to complete data analysis, qualitative data in the form of quotations from letters supplement the text. This volume and its data will provide nursing educators and administrators with the information they need to recruit and retain new students and employees.

FIGURE 1
Admissions to Basic RN Programs: 5-Year Trend

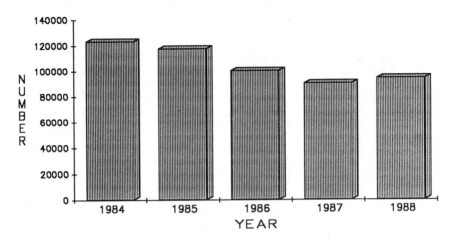

FIGURE 2
Newly Licensed Nurses by Type of Nursing Education

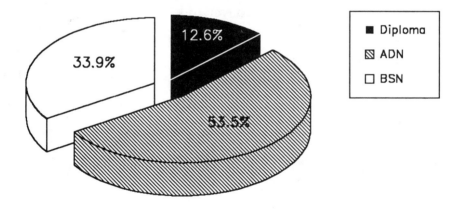

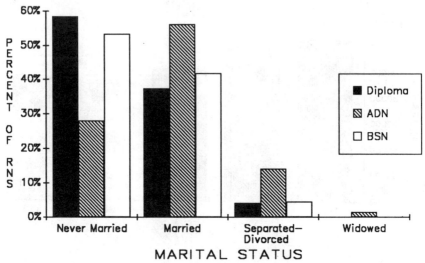

FIGURE 3
Marital Status of Newly Licensed Nurses by Program Type

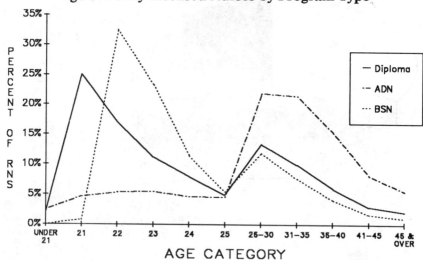

FIGURE 4
Age of Newly Licensed Nurses by Program Type

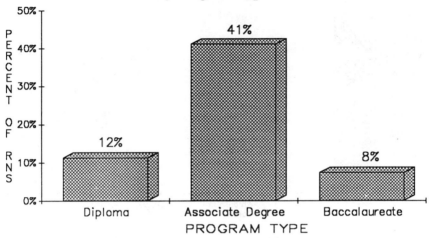

FIGURE 5
Prior LPN/LVN Licensure of Newly Licensed Nurses
by Program Type

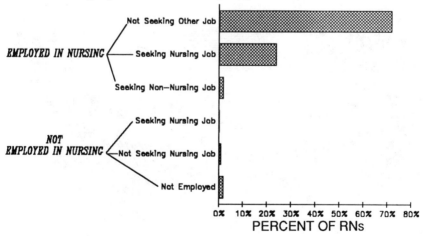

FIGURE 6
Employment Status of Newly Licensed Nurses

FIGURE 7
Employment Settings of Newly Licensed Nurses

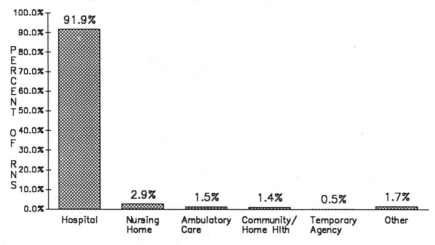

EMPLOYMENT SETTINGS

FIGURE 8
Mean Full-Time Salaries of Newly Licensed Nurses by Region

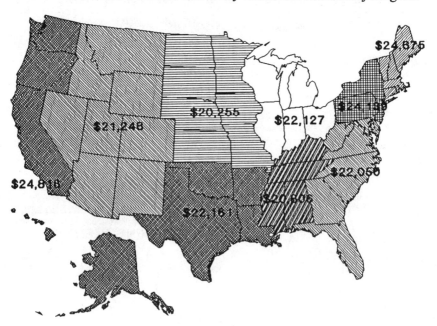

FIGURE 9
Job Satisfaction of Newly Licensed Nurses from
All Program Types

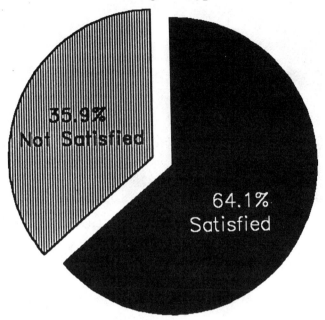

FIGURE 10
Main Source of Dissatisfaction with Employment

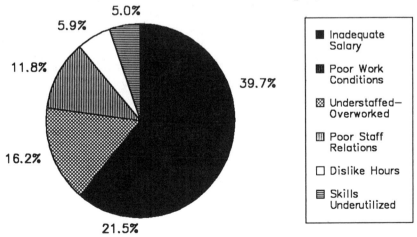

* Asked only of those 'not satisfied' with current employment (N=13,315)

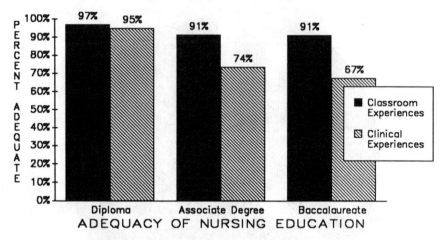

FIGURE 11
Adequacy of Nursing Education of Newly Licensed
Nurses by Program Type

3

PROFILE OF THE CONTEMPORARY NURSING POPULATION: FINDINGS FROM 1988 SAMPLE SURVEY OF REGISTERED NURSES DATA SOURCES

Evelyn B. Moses
Chief, Nursing Data and Analysis Staff,
Bureau of Health Professions,
Department of Health and Human Services
Washington, DC

In the mid-1970s, a methodological approach to obtaining data on the registered nurse population using sampling techniques was designed for the Division of Nursing of the Bureau of Health Professions in the U.S. Department of Health and Human Services. These studies, which are based on a sample of those who have current licenses to practice as registered nurses at the time of data collection, have been the main source of information on the country's registered nurses since 1977. The four studies that were carried out—September 1977, November 1980, November 1984, and March 1988—provide us with data on registered nurses over a span of about 10 years. They give us a profile of the nurses regardless of whether they are employed in nursing or not. They allow us to compare one segment of the population with another—hospital-employed nurses with those in community health—by their age, marital status, educational preparation, and salaries. And they provide us with data on trends over that decade.

FINDINGS OF THE 1988 SURVEY: HOW THE DATA COMPARES WITH 1977

The survey made in March 1988 came at a time when we were particularly concerned about nursing shortages. While presently it is generally thought that the shortages came about because the supply could not keep up with the demand rather than a decline in the supply itself, it is still important to know what the supply is and its characteristics. I will examine what the registered nurse population looks like now, as measured in March 1988, and look back to what it was like over the last 10 years to the present.

Numbers

When the initial concerns about the nursing shortage began to surface toward the end of 1986, it was difficult to convince people that, indeed, the supply of registered nurses had actually increased. Enrollments in schools of nursing had decreased (although the number graduating had not), hospitals were reporting high vacancies—obviously, the number of nurses had to have decreased. Further study and discussion brought about the conclusion that the supply had increased. This fact can be seen readily in Figure 1.

In March 1988, there were an estimated 2,033,032 individuals in the United States who had licenses to practice as registered nurses, 45% more than in September 1977. Of even more interest, though, the number of those who were employed in nursing increased at an even greater rate, with the highest increase occurring for the number employed full-time in nursing: There were 65% more registered nurses employed on a full-time basis in March 1988 than there were in September 1977. In March 1988, 1,099,576 of the 1,627,035 employed nurses were employed full-time.

Personal Characteristics

What do the 2 million registered nurses in the country look like? The registered nurse population has remained predominantly female. Although the number of men has increased along with the increase in the size of the total population, the proportion of that total that is male has changed from about 2% in 1977 to a little over 3% in 1988.

Registered nurses are predominantly white, nonHispanic. About 6% were from racial/ethnic minority backgrounds in 1977. Despite an increase in the number of nurses between 1984 and 1988, there was little change in the number of those with racial/ethnic minority backgrounds in 1988, when only 7.6% had such backgrounds.

In 1988, as in 1977, most registered nurses were married. In the September 1977 study it was estimated that 72% of all nurses were married and that 69% of those who were employed in nursing were married. In the 1988 study, the respective percentages were almost identical, 71 and 69.5, respectively.

It is interesting to note as well that a large portion of those who are married and have preschool age children are also part of the nurse labor force. In 1988, 82% of these registered nurses were employed in nursing, a proportion similar to that of all nurses. Eighty percent of all registered nurses were employed in nursing. The majority of nurses with young children, however, are part-timers. Over a third of all part-time nurses are married with preschool age children. One solution for the nursing shortage is to look toward part-time nurses providing more hours of work. In developing approaches to doing so, the needs of this relatively large group—those having young children—among the part-timers have to be taken into consideration.

As we look at the ages of the registered nurses there are changes that also have implications for future activities to solve nursing shortages. As Figure 2 shows, despite the increasing number of nurses in the population, there is a decline in those in the youngest age group. Since November 1980, when it was estimated that there were about 418,000 nurses who were less than 30 years old, that number has decreased by more than 100,000. In March 1988, there were an estimated 316,000 nurses under the age of 30. Thus, as you can see, the nurse population is getting older.

One of the major reasons for this is the older age at which individuals are graduating from basic nursing educational programs and thus entering into registered nurse licensure. In March 1988, those who had graduated within the past 5 years had a median age at graduation of 25, in contrast to a median age of 23 for those who had graduated between 5 and 10 years before that. Associate degree graduates are generally older than the others and their age level is increasing as well. The median age for the more recent associate degree graduates was 30 in contrast to a median of 27 for those who had graduated between 5 and 10 years ago.

However, while the increasing age level of nurses, is, in part, due to the older age at which students graduate these days, it is also related to the types of programs from which they are graduating. As Figure 3 shows, an increasingly higher proportion is coming from associate degree programs where large proportions of the older students are concentrated. Fifty-three percent of those who had graduated within the past 5 years were from such programs.

From the trends shown in these data, we can anticipate an increasing age level for registered nurses in the future. This has important implications for determining what the future supply of registered nurses might be. Although the activity rate at each age at any one given point in time is rather high—until you reach the oldest age groups—it still declines with age. About 97% of those who are less than 25 years old are employed in nursing while 70% of those who are in the 55–59 age group are employed in nursing.

Also, another of the solutions considered for the nursing shortage is to recruit from a much broader base of students: those who are older, already in the workforce and interested in changing careers, as well as those who are returning to the workforce. Obviously, this is a good approach to ensure that there are sufficient numbers of students in the face of increasing competition for students and a declining number of younger people from whom recruits can be obtained. At the same time, in determining what the future supply might be, recognition has to be given to the fact that, since they are starting in nursing at an older age, they will be a part of the nurse labor force for less time than would someone who might be younger.

An area which has shown substantial change over the time period during which these studies were being conducted is that of the educational preparation of the registered nurses. Figure 4 shows the distribution of the total registered nurse population according to basic nursing education received. Two very distinct trends are obvious. In 1977, those who had initially graduated from diploma programs made up three-quarters of the 1.4 million nurses at that time. By 1988, both the number and the proportion of these individuals had declined substantially. Some 990,000—or less than half of the 2 million nurses—were diploma graduates. The number of associate degree graduates, however, has grown rapidly in the time period, increasing from about 158,000, or 11% of the nurse population in 1977, to 576,000, or 28% of the nurse population in 1988. As I pointed out earlier, indications in the data are that these trends will continue into the future.

Of course, as we know, the determination of the educational preparation of the registered nurse has to take into account not only the initial education they bring to nursing but also the additional nursing-related education they achieve after becoming registered nurses. As Figure 5 indicates, the distribution of the registered nurses according to highest educational preparation also showed major changes since 1977. Here, too, we see the decline in diploma nurses and the increase in associate degree nurses. In addition, the proportion of the total population whose highest level of education was that of a baccalaureate degree increased from 18% in 1977 to 27% in 1988, and the proportion whose highest level was a master's degree or doctoral degree went from 4% to 6%. There were 557,000 nurses with baccalaureate degrees and 130,000 with master's degrees or doctorates in 1988. About 5,400 of the latter group had doctoral degrees.

Comparing the pace at which the registered nurse population obtains higher degrees beyond those with which they started out during the course of these surveys provides an interesting statistic. In each of the four studies, although the educational mix of the nurses showed substantial change, the proportion of the total nurse population who were enrolled in educational programs with nursing-related focus was about the same, about 10%. Of course, the number of those nurses increased each time since the population each time was larger.

Employment

Let us now look at those who are employed in nursing. Eight out of every 10 registered nurses were employed in nursing positions in March 1988. They numbered over 1.6 million. Both the proportion of those who were employed and the number employed were at the highest level when compared with the other studies in the series.

Figure 6 shows the distribution of the employed nurses in March 1988 arranged by their fields of employment. As has been the case in all the studies, the major place of employment is the hospital. Nurses working in the hospital setting numbered over 1.1 million, or 68% of the total employed, in March 1988. The number of those in hospital settings showed substantial increase over the course of the four studies. The 1988 total was 84% higher than that for 1977. Between November 1984 and March 1988, the number of nurses working in the hospital setting had increased about 93,000. I should point out here that these data include nurses who are working in the hospital through temporary employment services, unlike the figures given by Connie Adams in Chapter 1 which would relate specifically to those who are actually in the employ of the hospital. However, it is important to realize that, despite the decline in patient census and the expansion of nonhospital-based care, hospitals have been absorbing greater numbers and proportions of the registered nurse supply. Also, given that 2 of every 3 employed nurses are in hospitals, it would take vast changes in the distribution of health care sites for there to be a substantial shift in the proportional distribution of nursing positions between the hospital and the nonhospital setting.

Between 1984 and 1988 nurses working in ambulatory care settings increased about 29%, from about 97,000 to about 126,000. This increase was primarily due to changes in the numbers working in group practice physician offices, free-standing clinics and ambulatory surgery settings, and health maintenance organizations. The number of nurses in home health care also grew, with a 17% increase shown for those in nonhospital-based home health agencies. The growth in the numbers working in these settings was in sharp contrast to what happened in the nursing home setting. Between 1984 and 1988, there was a decline from an estimated 115,000 working in nursing homes and extended care facilities in 1984 to about 108,000 in March 1988. The number in 1988, however, represented a 35% increase over the number in 1977.

Salary

Salaries are an important issue when the nursing shortage is discussed. Many have pointed to the need to improve nursing salary levels to recruit into nursing and to retain those who are already in nursing. It has also been pointed out that more effective use could be made of registered nurses if nursing salaries were higher in comparison to other workers, thus making it more expensive to use nurses for functions better carried out by others who are paid less.

What has happened to nursing salaries over the decade in which these studies have been conducted? Figure 7 shows the average salary of a full-time employed nurse from each of the four studies in actual and "real" dollars. Real dollars take into account the effect of inflation on the value of money. These data show that the average annual salary of a full-time registered nurse between September 1977 and March 1988 more than doubled. In September 1977 it was $12,948; in March 1988, it was $28,383. In "real" earnings, however, the increase over that time was 16% and, as the figure shows, although the average actual salary was higher in 1980 than in 1977, in "real" dollar terms it had decreased during that period. Between November 1984, a time immediately preceding the shortage crisis, and March 1988, the average salary increased 21%. When inflation is discounted, the increase was 9%.

Since about two-thirds of the employed nurses were in staff-level positions, the average salary for staff nurses is an important measure of nursing salary levels. Full-time employed staff nurses averaged $26,263 in March 1988. This average, like that of all nurses, increased 21% since the 1984 study. A particular concern that has arisen in connection with the nursing shortage is that of the salary range to which a nurse could aspire during the course of a nursing career. One comparison concerning the average annual salary of the beginning nurse in National League for Nursing's Newly Licensed Nurse Survey, which is discussed by Peri Rosenfeld in Chapter 2, shows that the difference between what a beginning nurse makes and what the average is for all nurses in staff positions, regardless of how long they have been in nursing, is something less than $4,000.

As Figure 8 shows, in March 1988 staff nurses in occupational health settings and in hospitals had the highest average salaries among the various types of staff nurses, $27,389 and $27,196, respectively. Those in ambulatory care settings had the lowest—$21,528—followed by the staff nurses in nursing homes and other extended care facilities who averaged $22,381. Despite the relatively low average salary of those in nursing homes, between 1984 and 1988 that average salary increased 23%, a higher increase than in the other fields of nursing.

Geographic Distribution

Let us now take a brief look at how the registered nurse supply is distributed around the country. Because of large differences in population by state, comparisons are usually based on the ratio of nurses to population. Be cautioned, though, that these ratios should not be considered a measure of nursing services to the population since nurses most often work in a facility or some other type of organized nursing service. Therefore, to measure nursing services, the types of facilities and other organized nursing services that are located in a particular area need to be taken into account along with the number of nurses. On an overall basis, in the country as a whole, there were 668 employed registered nurses per 100,000 population in March 1988. As you can see in Figure 9, there was wide variation from state to state. Louisiana had the lowest ratio; 441 per 100,000 people. Massachusetts had the highest among the 50 states; 1,166 per 100,000 people. Generally, the ratios were lowest in the southern part of the country and highest in the northeastern part and in a portion of the north central area.

All states experienced gains in the number of employed nurses in the 10-year span of these surveys, as seen in Figure 10. However, the southern area, where the ratios were the lowest, generally showed the largest increases in the period. On the other hand, a number of the states with high ratios were among those on the low end of the scale.

SUMMARY

Although this might have seemed like a lot of data packed into a relatively short paper, this is but a part of the information available from the study. As I hope these statistics have demonstrated, the study provides answers to a number of questions surrounding the registered nurse population concerning quantity, quality, and the place of registered nurses within the health care services of the country.

FIGURE 1
Registered Nurse Population by Nursing Employment Status

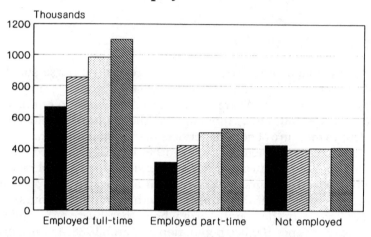

SOURCE: U.S. Department of Health and Human Services, Health Resources and Services Administration, Bureau of Health Professions, Division of Nursing. *The registered nurse population, findings from the National Sample Survey of Registered Nurses* (September 1977, November 1980, November 1984, March 1988). Washington, D. C.: Author.

FIGURE 2
Age Distribution of Registered Nurse Population: September 1977–March 1988

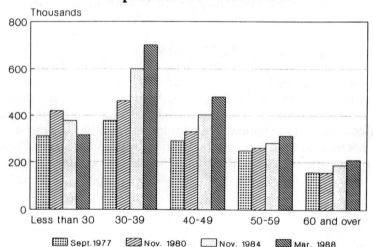

SOURCE: U.S. Department of Health and Human Services, Health Resources and Services Administration, Bureau of Health Professions, Division of Nursing. *The registered nurse population, findings from the National Sample Survey of Registered Nurses* (September 1977, November 1980, November 1984, March 1988). Washington, D. C.: Author.

FIGURE 3
Type of Basic Education of RNs by Year of Graduation: March, 1988

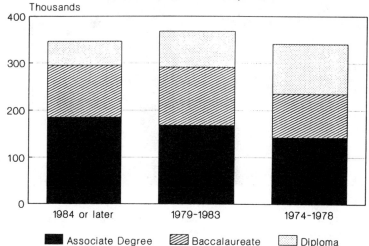

SOURCE: U.S. Department of Health and Human Services, Health Resources and Services Administration, Bureau of Health Professions, Division of Nursing. *The registered nurse population, findings from the National Sample Survey of Registered Nurses, March 1988.* Washington, D. C.: Author.

FIGURE 4
Basic Educational Preparation of Registered Nurses: September 1977–March 1988

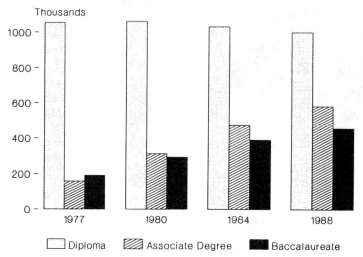

SOURCE: U.S. Department of Health and Human Services, Health Resources and Services Administration, Bureau of Health Professions, Division of Nursing. *The registered nurse population, findings from the National Sample Survey of Registered Nurses* (1977, 1980, 1984, 1988). Washington, D. C.: Author.

FIGURE 5
Highest Educational Preparation of Registered Nurses: September 1977–March 1988

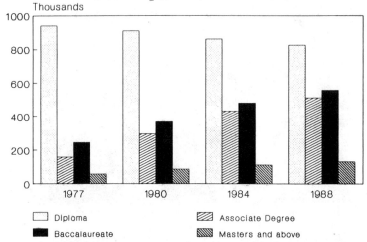

SOURCE: U.S. Department of Health and Human Services, Health Resources and Services Administration, Bureau of Health Professions, Division of Nursing. *The registered nurse population, findings from the National Sample Survey of Registered Nurses* (1977, 1980, 1984, 1988). Washington, D. C.: Author.

FIGURE 6
Field of Employment of Registered Nurses: March 1988

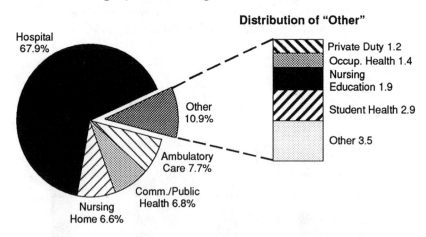

SOURCE: U.S. Department of Health and Human Services, Health Resources and Services Administration, Bureau of Health Professions, Division of Nursing. *The registered nurse population, findings from the National Sample Surveys of Registered Nurses, March 1988.* Washington, D. C.: Author.

FIGURE **7**

FIGURE **7**
Actual and "Real" Average Salaries of Full-Time Employed Registered Nurses

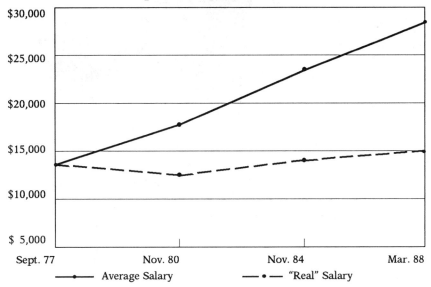

SOURCES: U.S. Department of Health and Human Services, Health Resources and Services Administration, Bureau of Health Professions, Division of Nursing. *The registered nurse population, findings from the National Sample Survey of Registered Nurses* (September 1977, November 1980, November 1984, March 1988). Washington, D.C.: Author. U.S. Department of Labor, Bureau of Labor Statistics. *Consumer price index*. Washington, D.C.: Author.

FIGURE **8**
Average Annual Earnings of Staff Nurses Employed Full Time by Field of Employment: November 1984 and March 1988

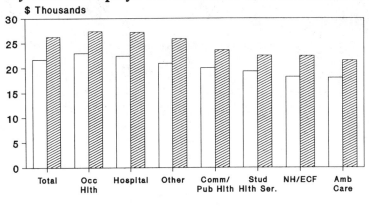

SOURCE: U.S. Department of Health and Human Services, Health Resources and Services Administration, Bureau of Health Professions, Division of Nursing. *The registered nurse population, findings from the National Sample Survey of Registered Nurses* (November 1984, March 1988). Washington, D.C.: Author.

FIGURE 9

Employed RNs Per 100,000 Population: March 1988

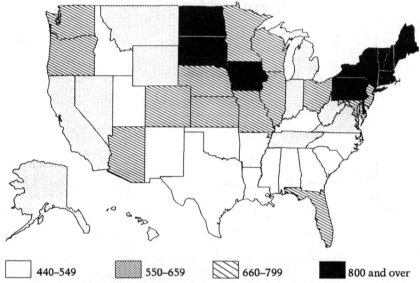

| | 440–549   550–659   660–799   800 and over

SOURCE: U.S. Department of Health and Human Services, Health Resources and Services Administration, Bureau of Health Professions, Division of Nursing. *The registered nurse population, findings from the National Sample Survey of Registered Nurses, March 1988*. Washington, D.C.: Author.

FIGURE 10

Percent Increase of Total Employed Registered Nurses: 1977–1988

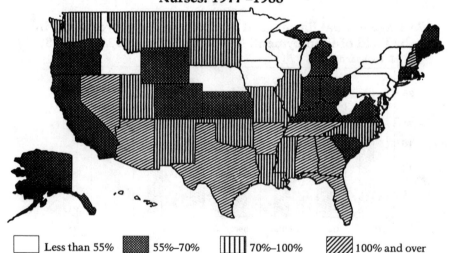

Less than 55%   55%–70%   70%–100%   100% and over

SOURCE: U.S. Department of Health and Human Services, Health Resources and Services Administration, Bureau of Health Professions, Division of Nursing. *The registered nurse population, findings from the National Sample Survey of Registered Nurses* (September 1977 and March 1988). Washington, D.C.: Author.

4

CHARACTERISTICS OF NEWLY LICENSED PRACTICAL/VOCATIONAL NURSE PRACTICE

Carolyn J. Yocom, PhD, RN
Director of Research Services
National Council of State Boards of Nursing
Chicago, Illinois

During the last several years, we have seen a number of changes occurring in the characteristics of health care recipients, levels of health care technology, and regulations affecting reimbursement for services. These have had an impact on the utilization of nursing personnel in all types of health care settings. Since others address the results of studies about registered nurses (see chapters by Adams, Moses, and Rosenfeld) this paper focuses on the Licensed Practical, or Vocational, Nurse (LPN/VN) and is based on the results of a job analysis study (Kane & Colton, 1988) performed by the National Council of State Boards of Nursing for the purpose of evaluating the validity of the licensing examination, NCLEX-PN.

SAMPLE CHARACTERISTICS AND RESPONSE RATES

The most recent job analysis study, published in June 1988, reflects data collected in January 1987 and January 1988 from two independent stratified random samples of LPN/VNs. The samples were drawn from the populations of individuals who were licensed as a result of successfully completing NCLEX-PN administered in October 1986 or October 1987. Stratification was based on the state where the licensing examination was administered. Information about sampling frames, sample sizes, and response rates are reported in Table 1.

DATA COLLECTION

The survey instrument used in this study, the *Survey of Nursing Activities*, was developed in 1984 for use in a role delineation study and a registered nurse (RN) job analysis study (Kane, Kingsbury, Colton, & Estes, 1986). The survey instrument permits the collection of information about characteristics of the work setting, the types of clients for whom the LPN/VN provides care, and the types of activities engaged in by newly licensed LPN/VNs.

Each of the newly licensed LPN/VNs in the two samples was sent a copy of the *Survey of Nursing Activities*, a postage-paid envelope, and a pencil. The packet also contained a cover letter from the president of the National Council describing the purposes and importance of the study, and asking for their participation. Approximately two weeks after the first mailing, a postcard reminder was sent to individuals who had not responded. After approximately two more weeks, a second copy of the questionnaire, return envelope, and pencil as well as a new cover letter from the president were sent to individuals who had still not responded. As reported in Table 1, response rates for the 1986 and 1987 groups were 64% and 54.7%, respectively. Following exclusion of data from respondents who reported they worked less than half-time in nursing or who did not provide usable data, the analysis files for the 1986 and 1987 groups consisted of responses from 885 and 870 individuals, respectively.

RESULTS

Selected results from the 1986–1987 job analysis study (Kane & Colton, 1988) describing the work environment of newly licensed LPN/VNs, the characteristics of their clients, and percentages of time newly licensed LPN/VNs spent on five major functions will be addressed.

Work Environment

Setting. Newly licensed LPN/VNs reported working in 23 different settings reflecting the three major health care delivery settings: acute care, long-term care, and ambulatory care. The distribution of individuals across these three major settings is reported in Table 2.

A comparison of the distributions for 1986 and 1987 revealed the occurrence of a shift in employment setting. In 1987, a greater percentage of respondents reported working in acute care and less in long-term care than in 1986. It is possible that this change may reflect the shortage of RNs and, therefore, more employment opportunities for LPN/VNs in acute care settings. Further examination of the data revealed that changes occurred primarily in two specific settings: medical-surgical units and skilled care facilities. In 1986, 19.9% (n = 167) of the respondents worked in medical-surgical nursing units and 19.1% (n = 169) worked in a skilled care facility. However, in 1987, 25.4% (n = 221) worked in medical-surgical nursing units and 16.2% (n = 141) worked in skilled care facilities. In contrast, there was less than a 1% change in the number of individuals working in any other specific acute care, long-term care, or ambulatory care setting.

Shift worked. There were substantial numbers of newly licensed LPN/VNs working on the day, evening, and night shifts and rotating shifts (see Table 3). However, the highest percentage of individuals, in both 1986 and 1987, worked evenings.

Client Characteristics

Client ages. Newly licensed LPN/VNs reported caring for clients of all ages (see Table 4). The most commonly indicated age group, in both 1986 (40.9%) and 1987 (37.2%), was "elderly clients." An additional 29.7% (1986) and 32.2% (1987) indicated they worked with two different age groups, "adults (ages 15–65)" and "elderly clients." The only other age group identified by a large percentage of respondents was "adults (ages 15–65)." Since the majority of respondents reported they worked in medical-surgical nursing units or long-term care facilities, these findings are not surprising. In addition, the two most common age groups identified by respondents working in clients' homes were "elderly clients" or a combination of "adults" and "elderly clients."

Client health problems/conditions. As indicated in Table 5, a large number of respondents indicated they cared for clients with a broad range of acuity ("multiple/other" category) (1986: 68.2%; 1987: 60.1%). Of the individual choices, "clients with stabilized chronic conditions" were the most frequently identified by both groups (1986: 12.5%; 1987: 16.2%).

Nursing Functions

Both 1986 and 1987 respondents reported they spent the majority of their time providing direct ("hands-on") patient care (78.7% and 79%, respectively) and indirect (planning, charting, consulting, etc.) patient care (11.5% and 11.1%, respectively). In addition, small but significant amounts of time were spent in management/administrative activities (1986: 4.9%; 1987: 5%). Table 6 provides the percentages of time (1986 and 1987 data combined) devoted to five functional areas, by type of work setting. As can be seen, the setting in which the newly licensed LPN/VN worked had an impact on the percentage of time devoted to direct and indirect client care activities and to management/administrative activities. Given the staffing patterns in long-term care facilities, it was not surprising that respondents working in these settings reported a greater percentage of time devoted to management (7.8%) and indirect care (16.1%) than those in other settings. This finding is supported by information obtained in response to the question, "Are you a charge nurse or an assistant head nurse?" As seen in Table 7, 72% of all respondents working in long-term care facilities indicated that they assumed charge nurse or assistant head nurse responsibilities. However, neither the scope nor the frequency of assuming these responsibilities was assessed.

CONCLUSIONS

When the results of this study are compared with the outcomes of a previous job analysis study (Ference, 1983) commissioned by the National Council of State Boards of Nursing, they indicate that changes have occurred in the practice settings and types of clients cared for by newly licensed LPN/VNs. The 1986–1987 data indicate that the new LPN/VN cares for an older group of clients than previously reported and that a greater number of these clients are cared for in long-term care facilities as opposed to acute care settings. However, newly licensed LPN/VNs in long-term care facilities devoted less time to the provision of direct care to clients and more time engaged in the provision of indirect care and management activities than their counterparts in acute care facilities.

REFERENCES

Ference, H. (1983). *Practical nurse role delineation and validation study for the National Council Licensure Examination for Practical Nurses.* Monterey, CA: CTB/McGraw-Hill.

Kane, M., & Colton, D. (1988). *Job analysis of newly-licensed practical/ vocational nurses: 1986–1987.* Chicago: National Council of State Boards of Nursing.

Kane, M., Kingsbury, C., Colton, D., & Estes, C. (1986). *A study of nursing practice and role delineation and job analysis of entry-level performance of registered nurses.* Chicago: National Council of State Boards of Nursing.

TABLE 1

Sampling Frames, Sample Sizes, and Response Rates for 1986 and 1987 LPN/VN Job Analysis Studies

	1986	1987
Sampling frame	20,456	18,896
Sample size	3,415	3,153
Number returned	2,074	1,654
Response rate, %	64.0	54.7

TABLE 2

Distribution of Newly Licensed Practical/Vocational Nurses, by Type of Work Setting

Setting	1986		1987	
	n	%	*n*	%
Acute care	197	22.3	271	26.7
Long-term care	289	32.7	252	30.8
Ambulatory	79	8.9	60	7.9
Multiple	320	36.2	287	34.6

TABLE 3

Distribution of Newly Licensed Practical/Vocational Nurses, by Shift Worked

Shift	1986		1987	
	n	%	*n*	%
Days	243	27.6	208	24.0
Evenings	280	31.8	248	28.7
Nights	179	20.3	204	23.6
Rotating	152	17.3	180	20.8
Other/multiple	27	3.0	25	2.9

TABLE 4
**Ages of Clients Cared for by Newly Licensed Practical/
Vocational Nurses**

Age Group	1986		1987	
	n	%	*n*	%
Newborns	2	0.2	2	0.2
Children/infants	10	1.1	8	0.9
Adults (15–65)	140	15.8	142	16.3
Elderly (over 65)	362	40.9	324	37.2
Newborns/children/infants	5	0.6	6	0.7
Newborns/adults	16	1.8	11	1.3
Newborns/elderly	0	—	2	0.2
Children/infants/adults	20	2.3	17	2.0
Children/infants/elderly	6	0.7	6	0.7
Adults/elderly	263	29.7	280	32.2
Multiple/other	61	6.9	72	8.3

TABLE 5
**Acuity/Condition of Clients Cared for by Newly Licensed
Practical/Vocational Nurses**

Acuity/Condition	1986		1987	
	n	%	*n*	%
Well clients	31	3.5	32	3.7
Maternity clients	17	1.9	10	1.1
Chronic conditions	111	12.5	141	16.2
Acute conditions	76	8.6	99	11.4
Terminally ill	19	2.1	22	2.5
Behavioral disorders	27	3.1	29	3.3
Multiple/other	604	68.2	501	60.1

TABLE 6
**Percentage of Time Spent on Five Major Functions by Newly
Licensed Practical/Vocational Nurses, by Type of Work Setting**

Function	Setting		
	Acute	Long-term	Ambulatory
Administration	1.6	7.8	5.3
Direct client care	88.9	71.3	78.1
Indirect client care	6.0	16.1	10.0
Education of students	0.9	1.3	1.3
Research	2.1	2.7	2.4
Other	0.6	0.9	2.8

TABLE 7

Distribution of Newly Licensed Practical/Vocational Nurses Indicating They Were a Charge Nurse or Assistant Head Nurse, by Type of Setting

Setting	Yes		No	
	n	%	*n*	%
Acute care (*n* = 465)	7	1.5	458	98.5
Long-term care (*n* = 536)	386	72.0	150	28.0
Ambulatory care (*n* = 138)	22	16.5	116	83.5

Nursing Centers

5

COSTS AND REVENUE SOURCES FOR NURSING CENTERS

Norman D. Brown, EdD, RN
Associate Professor of Nursing
The University of Arkansas
at Little Rock College for Medical Sciences
Member, Executive Committee
NLN Council for Nursing Centers

Nursing centers are nurse owned and operated enterprises which provide basic health and human services. The types of activities conducted by these enterprises ranges from a one-nurse consulting firm to the multifaceted university-based academic nursing centers. I focus on two elements to be considered in the planning and implementation of nursing centers: (1) cost estimates and (2) potential sources of revenue. The information presented is based upon my personal experience as the director of an academic nursing center and information gained through conducting doctoral student research on the evolution of nursing centers (Barger, 1986; Brown, 1988). This chapter presents practical information and addresses the reader as a potential nurse entrepreneur or academician who is studying the feasibility of establishing a nursing center.

COSTS

Research and Development

Research. Time and talent are essential elements in the planning and implementation of a nursing center. The establishment of any health and human service requires an in-depth assessment of the current status of existing services and the need for new services and/or the augmentation of existing services. This means that to be successful your nursing center will be designed to provide products and services in areas where there are service "gaps" in your local health system—or you may be able to supplement existing services which are overutilized. In order to identify these target populations as opportunities to provide service, you must conduct a marketing study which includes the following:

- A demographic analysis of the region to be served.

- An assessment of existing health and human services in your region (noting strengths and weaknesses).

- An assessment of your assets and limitations.

- An assessment of potential funding sources.

Conducting a solid research and development study can require as long as a year or more. Key resources for this type of information will be the nursing directors of hospitals, faculty of nursing education programs, and nursing directors of local and state health and human service agencies. Additional technical assistance in the development of a business plan, marketing scheme, and plan of operation can be obtained through collaboration with faculty and students in college and university schools of business. These types of academic programs will often have students who are pursuing advanced degrees and who are required to develop marketing, business research, and development projects.

Development and Implementation. Once a health or human service need that you wish to address has been identified, you will need to consider the elements of a nursing center that will be the manifestation of your service. Assuming you or someone you can recruit are fully qualified to provide the service, there are many components, or elements, which must be considered in detail. These elements include:

- *Protocols*: These should include policies and procedures for clinical services, quality assurance, and financial accounting methods that can be self-developed or developed with the assistance of consultation.

- *Salary-compensation packages*: Cost factors will vary by regions. Generally, these costs will include the salary for each person employed by the project plus 25–35% for fringe benefits.

- *Space requirements*: Again, this element will depend on the types of services to be provided and the desired location of the proposed nursing center. Commercial property will usually be priced by the amount of square footage required, ease of access, parking space available, and proximity to other businesses.

- *Specialized equipment*: Consider lease/lease purchase agreements for specialized equipment you cannot acquire through manufacturer donation and/or purchase plans. It is possible to "share" equipment between similar projects at various sites to avoid duplication in equipment inventories.

- *Security*: Protection of vital records and specialized equipment should be assured through the use of some form of burglary and fire detection alarm systems. These services may come with the commercial property or they may have to be installed. Property insurance to protect your project against disastrous losses must be considered.

- *Systematic record keeping system*: Computer-based data management systems are affordable, reliable, and can provide excellent data bases for program evaluation/research. Again, consider lease/lease purchase of these systems with some form of data backup in case of disaster.

- *Liability insurance*: Note that, in most cases, academic nursing centers can use their institutional liability insurance and/or institutional immunity to cover their activities. This type of arrangement is a true asset in the development and implementation of an academic nursing center. Each insurance package will have a price based upon the types of services and the amount of coverage you wish to provide.

Perseverance and resourcefulness will serve you well as you establish these fiscal elements of your nursing center.

REVENUE SOURCES

Many, if not most, academic nursing centers are supported in large part by their parent institutions through general operating funds. Faculty time ultimately translates into money for academic administrators. Many academic nursing centers are established as "pilot services" which, once their efficacy is established, are able to develop service contracts with local and state agencies for continued growth. Health and human services that are currently rich in contract funding include prenatal care, geriatric case management, teen pregnancy interventions, indigent and homeless health care, and "caregivers" support.

Depending upon your state and local regulations, reimbursement for nursing center services may be sought from Medicare and Medicaid. Private insurance carriers may also honor billing statements from nursing centers. However, it is advisable to contact each carrier regarding this matter prior to the delivery of services. At the state and local level, funds may be available through a variety of agencies. State agencies dealing with health and human services are frequently searching for cost-effective service delivery contractors. At the local level, governmental officials should be approached regarding the use of Community Development Block Grants to support nursing centers in medically underserved neighborhoods. Many churches and private philanthropic foundations can be approached to support nursing center activities targeting selected populations.

Funds to support demonstration projects are limited; however, the Robert Wood Johnson Foundation, Kellogg Foundation, Ford Foundation, and others are exploring the potential contributions of nurse-managed health service delivery models. The Health Care Finance Administration, the USPHS Division of Nursing, and National Center for Nursing Research are also entertaining the development of these types of activities. Also, at the federal level, the Older Americans Act of 1987 and the parallel 1988 Title II regulations encourage Councils of Governments and Area Agencies on Aging to develop prototype health education and promotion programs. Significant funds are becoming available for the development of nursing centers, particularly in rural and other medically underserved areas. These types of funds are well suited to service delivery development and research in nursing center service delivery models.

In conclusion, this discussion has highlighted many of the elements related to the costs and resources to be considered in the development of a nursing center. Unique considerations for each nursing center may not have been covered here and this is only one point of reference for the development of these types of health service delivery systems. The well-planned nursing center will be developed around nursing expertise and will be "demographically driven," i.e., serving well-defined target populations. Diverse funding sources will need to be explored, with nurses themselves providing most, if not all, of the venture capital, time, and talent to develop meaningful products and services. The profession of nursing has evolved to the point where nursing centers are viable, cost effective, and essential health and human services. Whether academically based or individual enterprises, the nursing center concept could be the most dynamic health and human service innovation in the history of our modern health care system.

SELECTED READINGS

Atton, D. M. (1980). A nursing clinic: The challenge for student learning opportunity. *Journal of Nursing Education, 19*, 153–158.

Barger, S. E. (1986). Personnel issues in academic nursing centers. *Nurse Educator*, 3:26–29.

Barger, S. E. (1986). Academic nursing centers: A demographic profile. *Journal of Professional Nursing, 2,* 246–251.

Berdie, D. R. (1986). *Questionnaires: Design and use.* Metuchen, NJ: Scarecrow Press.

Brown, N. D. (1986). Shaping clinical practice in community health nursing. In M. Assay (Ed.), *Proceedings of the National Community Health Nursing Conference,* (pp. 117–145). Chapel Hill: University of North Carolina.

Brown, N. D. (1988). The current administrative practices of academic nursing centers in N.L.N. accredited schools of nursing. Ann Arbor, MI: University Microfilms International, Dissertation Information Service.

Collison, C. R. (1980). Is practice a viable faculty role? *Nursing Outlook, 28,* 677–679.

Curan, R., & Riley, D. W. (1984). Faculty practice plans: Will they work? *Nursing Economics, 2,* 316–323.

Diers, D. (1980). *Faculty practice: Models, methods, and madness.* New York: National League for Nursing.

Dolan, J. (1978). *Nursing in society: A historical perspective.* Philadelphia: Saunders.

Flatt, M. M., & Blecke, J. (1983). Scarce clinical facilities? Not in community health. *Michigan Nurse, 1,* 8–9.

Free, T. (1983). Faculty practice in primary care. *Nursing Outlook, 33,* 192–194.

Grimes, D. (1980). Meeting the health care needs of the elderly through a community nursing center. *Nursing Administration Quarterly, 4,* 31–40.

Gunn, I. P. (1986). Nursing innovations help reach traditional goals. *Nursing Health and Care, 7,* 353–362.

Hauf, B. (1985). An evaluative study of a nursing center for community health nursing student experience. *Journal of Nursing Education, 16,* 11–17.

Henrich, J. (1984). Guidelines for community based nursing services. Kansas City: American Nurses' Association.

Infante, M. S. (1986). The conflicting roles of nurse and nurse educator. *Nursing Outlook, 34,* 94–96.

Isaac, S., & Michael, W. B. (1982). *Handbook in research and evaluation* (2nd ed). San Diego: Edits Publishers.

Jezek, J. (1981). Economic realities of faculty practice. *National League for Nursing Publication, 15,* 18–31.

Johnson Foundation, R. W. (1987). Health care for the uninsured. *Quarterly Report, 3,* 1–8.

Jolly, P., & Smith, W. P. (1981). *Medical practice plans in 1980.* Washington, DC: Association of American Medical Colleges.

Jones, A. (1973). Nursing centers for health services, *JNYSNA,* 4:1:33.

Kuhn, J. K. (1985). Faculty practice: A philosophical issue for the '80's. *Texas Nursing, 10,* 11–15.

Labaw, P. J. (1980). *Advanced questionnaire design.* Cambridge, MA: Abbott Books.

Langford, T. L. (1982). *Managing and being managed.* Englewood Cliffs, NJ: Prentice Hall.

Lavin, K. (1947). Frontiers in group dynamics: Concepts, methods, and reality in social science. *Human Relations, 1,* 5–42.

Millonig, V. L. (1986). Faculty practice: A view of its development, benefits, and barriers. *Journal of Professional Nursing, 3,* 166–171.

Morgan, B. S., et al. (1984). An experience in health planning for baccalaureate nursing students. *Public Health Nursing, 1,* 168–173.

Nettles-Carlson, B. (1987). Group faculty practice: Dream vs. reality. *Nurse Educator, 5,* 8–12.

Ossler, C. C. (1982). Establishment of a clinic for faculty and student clinical practice. *Nursing Quarterly, 30,* 402–405.

Putt, A. M. (1978). *General systems theory applied to nursing.* Boston: Little, Brown.

Scheffler, R. M. (1980). Review of the economic evidence for prevention. *Medical Care, 5,* 473–484.

Selby, T. (1984). Nurse managed centers show their potential. *American Nurse, 16,* 1–10, 19.

Stanhope, M. (1985) *Community health nursing.* New York: Mosby.

Stone, D. A. (1979). Health care cost containment. *Journal of Health Politics, Policy, and Law, 4,* 176–199.

Sudman, S. (1982). *Asking questions.* San Francisco: Jossey-Bass.

Tornay, R. (1987). Toward faculty practice. *Journal of Nursing Education, 1,* 137.

Texas Department of Health. (1987). Indigent Health Care Programs. *Annual Report.* Austin: Author.

Volpe, L., & Sperry, B. (1987). The Texas Indigent Health Care and Treatment Act: Initial implementation assessment. Austin: Texas Department of Human Services: Office of Strategic Management, Research, and Development.

6

NURSING CENTERS—STATE OF THE ART AND FUTURE INITIATIVES: SERVICES AND MARKETING STRATEGIES

Elizabeth Holman, MS, RN
Health Services Coordinator
Community Health Services
Scottsdale, Arizona

Services and marketing are dependent upon each other. One cannot exist without the other. The services provided by nursing centers may be of the highest quality and may fulfill a need of the community; however, if those services are not adequately marketed, they are wasted! Conversely, the most sophisticated marketing program will be unsuccessful if the products or services being marketed do not meet the needs of the community.

Services offered by nursing centers in the United States generally focus on health promotion activities such as health education classes, health screenings, and physical assessments. These services are being offered at various sites, such as university campuses, senior centers, churches, and freestanding centers.

Outreach activities such as cholesterol screenings are being offered in schools, health fairs, industrial complexes, small businesses, and government entities. Additional screenings such as blood pressure, glucose, and triglycerides are sometimes offered in conjunction with cholesterol.

Health education classes appear to be popular services offered by staff of nursing centers. Subjects vary and can include topics of interest to new parents, teenagers, and the elderly. In addition, health teaching is being offered to groups of employees at work places.

Women's health care has been identified by some nursing centers as a *natural service*. After all, women make 25% more office visits than men after age 14 (Triolo, 1987). Women not only are the largest group of consumers of health care but they are also the health care managers of their families.

Additional services offered throughout the country include developmental testing of children, immunizations, influenza injections, school and camp physical examinations, weight control programs, treatment of minor illnesses, and home health care.

Are nursing centers meeting the needs of communities with these services? Should the services of nursing centers be expanded? In 1985–86 the six most common diagnoses identified by the national center for health care statistics included essential hypertension, normal pregnancy, health supervision of infants and children, otitis media, general medical examinations, and acute respiratory infections (McLemore & Delozier, 1987). Are we competing with the medical community for clientele with the above diagnoses?

The health care marketplace has seen profound changes in recent years. Traditional health care providers are becoming accustomed to considerable competition (Auttonberry, 1988). Nurses are recognizing, as are health care administrators, that utilization of marketing concepts now means *survival*, especially in a nonprofit organization. In addition, internal and external forces influencing nursing are cause for concern for the entire profession. These forces are:

1. Increasing aging population

2. Escalating health care costs

3. Oversupply of physicians

4. Technological advancements

5. Increased emphasis on health promotion and self-care

All these trends suggest what health care services are being required by consumers and, more importantly, whom they will seek to provide these services. Marketing services is an honorable discipline that utilizes scientific tools and it is an optional management system that can sustain organizations. (It is okay to market nursing services.)

I would like to discuss six components that should be considered when developing a marketing plan (Adams, Hockema, & Wood, 1988). As I discuss these components, I will give examples from my experience in marketing programs at our nursing center.

MISSION STATEMENT OF THE ORGANIZATION

The mission statement should be a broad philosophical statement that denotes the parameters in which marketing plans can be developed.

Example: The nursing model of health care is appropriately focused on the promotion of health and wellness as well as on providing care of minor illnesses and referral service.

Internal-External Analysis

A. *Internal*

1. Analysis of present services: Women's health and treatment of minor illnesses were the most frequently used services of our nursing center.

2. Fees for services: Our fees were more reasonable than fees being charged by physicians in the area. For instance, our fee for a woman's health exam is $45, including lab work.

3. Staffing: Our staff is adequate; staff is enthusiastic and willing to try new ideas and offer new services. Staff wants the clinic to succeed.

B. *External analysis revealed*

1. Analysis of services being offered by other health care providers: There are several urgent care centers within a radius of one-half mile to five miles of the center. There are also some private physicians' offices within a five-mile vicinity.

2. Analysis of clients who utilize the clinic regarding insurance policies: There are variances among insurance carriers. Approximately 25% of the clientele using our center have insurance.

3. Correlation of life-threatening illnesses, such as heart disease, some cancers, and AIDS, to life style: Health education and counseling to individuals and groups is becoming more important.

4. Federal and state controls have direct influence on health care today: The indigents in Arizona receive state health care while the more affluent have the funding to pay private physicians. Our target group, therefore, became those individuals who could not afford private health care and were not classified by the state as indigents.

SETTING OBJECTIVES

These objectives must be congruent with the organization's daily operation—its history—and its mission and goals.

Example: Our staff decided to "market" women's health. Marketing women's health certainly paralleled our mission statement—that of promoting health and wellness.

Our objectives were:

1. To provide reasonable, quality health care for women
2. To provide a convenient time for women to receive health care
3. To increase clinic clientele
4. To increase the awareness of the general public about Community Health Services Clinic

DEVELOPING ACTION STRATEGY

Start by assigning one staff member to be responsible for the center's marketing program. This is when the marketing objectives are translated into a plan for specific action. Use marketing consultants or marketing students from your university school of business if necessary.

Example: Our budget was low for advertising; therefore, we depended on public service announcements in newspapers, radio, and television. We designed flyers with the help of a nearby Kwik-Kopy graphic artist. The flyers were then photocopied at the College of Nursing and distributed to houses and apartments in the proximity of the clinic, public library, and clinic reception room. Flyers were taken to business sites by the cholesterol screening team.

INTEGRATION OF PLANS

Much of this integration begins immediately during planning since staff members need to provide input while developing the strategy.

Example: Our women's health program became an integral part of the total program being offered by the nursing center. In addition to the exam itself, staff members began classes on family planning, lactation, menopause, and prenatal classes.

EVALUATION AND FEEDBACK

Example: What marketing strategies worked best? How did women find out about our services? Which strategies should be expanded and which should be eliminated?

To answer these questions, we devised a short questionnaire that was given to all new clients by the receptionist. Periodically, the women's health program was evaluated by staff, and changes were made accordingly.

The marketing process provides an effective management system in which planning is driven by a perceived demand. Implementation results from a documented need, and evaluation occurs through the ongoing measurement of meaningful results. Nurse executives can cultivate skills in marketing simply by remembering the *four Ps*: product, promotion, place, and price (Stanton & Stanton, 1988).

PROJECTIONS FOR THE FUTURE

1. Increase services. In addition to health promotion services, offer treatment of minor illness and referrals. Nursing centers are sometimes limited because of the limited perceptions of those in charge. Too many are afraid to go out on a limb to increase services.

2. Implement a fair-fee policy. Do not be reluctant to charge for services.

3. Identify target populations.

4. Keep statistics. Document the value of nursing services.

5. Continue Research and Evaluation.

6. HMO membership. Investigate possibility of becoming a member of a health maintenance organization (HMO) or a preferred provider member of an insurance plan.

The new Secretary of the U.S. Department of Health and Human Services, Dr. Louis W. Sullivan, has targeted health promotion as one of the top priorities for his agency. In recent public statements, Dr. Sullivan has stressed the cost effectiveness of preventive medicine and health education and has said his agency would provide federal support for local and private initiatives to combat preventable diseases.

Nursing centers have already been doing what Dr. Sullivan intends to do—we make our communities aware of our services by implementing marketing strategies so that we not only survive but also thrive.

REFERENCES

Adams, G.A., Hockema, M.L., & Wood, L. (1988). Integrating marketing into nursing service. *Nursing Management, 19*(9), 30–34.

Auttonberry, D.S. (1988). The emerging role of the master's-prepared nurse in marketing. *Nursing Management, 19*(9), 40–43.

McLemore, T., & Delozier, J. (1987). 1985 summary: National ambulatory medical care survey. *NCHS Advanced Data, 28.*

Stanton, M., & Stanton, G. (1988). Marketing nursing: A model for success. *Nursing Management, 19*(9), 36–38.

Triolo, P.K. (1987). Marketing women's health care. *Journal of Nursing Administration, 17*(11), 10–15.

7

HEALING AND WHOLENESS: A CASE STUDY OF A NURSE-MANAGED AIDS CENTER

Janet M. Smerke, PhD, RN
Assistant Professor of Nursing
University of Texas at Tyler
Tyler, Texas

The presence of the human immunodeficiency virus (HIV) and acquired immunodeficiency syndrome (AIDS) have become fatal diagnoses for an increasing number of persons. Clients with HIV-related infections are desperately seeking competent and compassionate care for their illnesses. Yet, even today, there remain limited services and facilities available to these persons and their significant others. In addition, there are a limited number of nurses who are actively involved in competently and compassionately facilitating their care regimes.

EPIDEMIOLOGY OF AIDS

According to the World Health Organization's AIDS update, the number of persons with HIV infections and AIDS worldwide increased by 40% in a 9-month period ending April 30, 1989. The world total increase was 151,790 persons. The Americas had the highest numerical increase, yet the region as a whole had a 34% increase, the lowest percentage of increase. The highest percentage of increase was experienced by Europe with a 68% increase ("Worldwide number," 1989).

The total number of infected persons reported by the U.S. Centers for Disease Control as of April 13, 1989 was 89,501 persons, which represented a 29.5% increase. The prevalence of HIV/AIDS and the proportional distribution of cases among high-risk populations in the United States is: 61% are homosexual/bisexual males, 20% are IV drug abusers, 7% are homosexual IV drug users, 4% are heterosexual cases, 3% are transfusion/blood components, 3% are undetermined cases, 1% are hemophilia/coagulation disorders, and 1% are children born from an AIDS parent ("Worldwide number," 1989). In contrast, the prevalence of HIV/AIDS and the proportional distribution of cases among high-risk populations in Colorado is: 76% are homosexual/bisexual males, 11% are homosexual IV drug users, 5% are IV drug abusers, 3% are hemophilia/coagulation disorders, 3% are transfusion/blood components, 2% are undetermined cases, 1% are heterosexual cases, and .10% are children born from an AIDS parent ("HIV/AIDS monthly," 1989).

The Colorado Department of Health ("HIV/AIDS monthly," 1989) reported that as of May 30, 1989, Colorado had 1,027 confirmed cases of AIDS and ranked 17th in the nation for the number of AIDS cases reported. Anderson (1988) reported that new cases of AIDS in Colorado are being diagnosed at the rate of 22 per month and this increase is in pace with the national rate. For each confirmed case of AIDS, there are at least 15 to 22 persons who are HIV positive (CDC, 1988). Eighty-five percent of the cases have been identified in the Denver metropolitan area, yet the infection is also spreading to the outlying regions of the state.

Over 40% (411) of the clients with AIDS in Colorado have been identified either at the Veterans Administration Medical Center, Denver (DVAMC); Denver Department of Health and Hospitals (DDHH); or University Hospital (UH). Estimates suggest that up to 50-60% of the 1,027 clients with AIDS in Colorado have received on-going medical care at the three institutions, since clients often move into public institutions when their financial resources are expended. Further, additional persons with HIV-related infections are followed at each institution. Current caseload of persons with HIV-related infections (HIV positive and AIDS) at the three institutions is approximately 450 clients.

COURSE OF HIV INFECTION

If the infection with HIV progresses to a symptomatic stage, the incubation period ranges from about 6 months to 8 years or more. The mean incubation period of AIDS is now estimated at greater than 7 years (Institute of Medicine, 1988). Early symptoms may include tiredness, fever, loss of appetite and weight, diarrhea, sweats, and swollen lymph nodes usually in the neck, axillae, or groin.

The diagnosis of AIDS depends upon the presence of certain opportunistic infections plus a positive serum test for the antibody to HIV. Persons who develop AIDS are at risk for a broad spectrum of opportunistic infections and cancers. Clients with AIDS usually suffer from several of these infections. AIDS clients are also at risk for a number of cancers such as Kaposi's sarcoma and lymphomas. Additionally, HIV infection also directly affects the central nervous system. At some point during their illness at least 65% of those with AIDS will develop some degree of neurologic deficit, ranging from mild memory loss to fulminant presenile dementia. Average survival after diagnosis with AIDS is 2 years, although evidence indicates that zidovudine (AZT) has decreased 1-year morbidity from approximately 33% to 10% (Institute of Medicine, 1988).

COST OF CARE

The current projections are that the medical care costs for AIDS in the United States in 1991 will be $8 to $16 billion, not considering the rather sizable bill for the health care needs of clients with other conditions within the spectrum of HIV-related infections (Institute of Medicine and National Academy of Sciences, 1986). Costs in the next decade could be in the tens of billions of dollars (Koop, 1987). The most cost-effective way to manage HIV infections is in noninstitutional settings (Droste, 1987; Smith, 1987). In addition, noninstitutional settings foster the environment of ability-focused rather than disability-focused care that is preferred by clients and families. Also important to any plan for AIDS care is coordination of services among various levels of care and among the social and health care professionals who provide economic and health care support to clients (McCaffrey, 1987).

TRENDS IN HEALING MODALITIES

Need for Client Care

Ninety-four percent of the care required by persons with HIV-related infections is nursing care (Presidential Commission on the Human Immunodeficiency Virus Epidemic, 1988). This care begins with counseling of persons who are having serologic testing for the antibodies to HIV. There is evidence that health promoting behaviors such as healthy nutrition, minimizing reexposure to the virus, and avoidance of nicotine and other recreational drugs may slow the course of the infections (Hay, 1986, 1988). Thus, even in the asymptomatic phases of the infection, nurses can help and empower persons with HIV-related infections and their significant others to focus on the positive options available, rather than on anxiety and despair.

Many of the early symptoms of HIV-related infections are amenable to traditional hygienic, nutritional, and supportive nursing interventions. This care is time consuming and requires individualized approaches that take into account unique daily activities, ability to make significant behavioral changes, and variable responses. Additionally, complementary caring modalities such as the transpersonal caring process, massage, therapeutic touch, meditation, imagery/visualization, and crystals and candles have been effective in symptom management for clients with HIV-related infections (Hay, 1986, 1988; Matthews-Simonton, Simonton, & Creighton, 1984; Serinus, 1987; Siegel, 1986). Educational and emotional support are increasingly required by clients and their significant others as the infection becomes symptomatic. Family caregivers may need instruction in physical care and interventions to relieve the burden posed by the physical, cognitive, and emotional effects of the infection. Bereavement support for individuals with HIV-related infections and their significant others is a long-term and ongoing process as they recognize and come to terms with the potential or actual outcome of the disease. Counseling and emotional support by trained psychiatric clinical nurse specialists combat the high stress levels, isolation, sadness, and depression common among these clients. Although the symptoms and responses to the disease may be mild or intense, most clients express preference for the emphasis on hope, meaning in the experience, maintenance of a normal and high-quality way of life, and empowerment to identify options and make choices about their care (Goff & McDonough, 1986; O'Brien, Oerlemans-Buan, & Blanchfield, 1987). The importance of accommodating these preferences continues even when the progression of the underlying HIV-related infection and secondary opportunistic infections and cancers necessitate rigorous medical therapy.

In summary, most of the care required by persons with HIV-related infections is nursing care. This care is best delivered in a noninstitutional setting with a prevention and wellness-focused milieu. A broad spectrum of nursing services is needed, encompassing the care, cure, and coordination functions of nursing, and ranging from high technology drug administration to psychoemotional support; from traditional basic hygienic nursing to complementary caring modalities. In 1987 an analysis of services available to persons with HIV-related infections in the Denver metropolitan area revealed a dearth of noninstitutional alternatives with available community-based care being used to maximal capacity (Smerke, 1988). Gaps were noted in the areas of education, health promotion, counseling, and emotional support for persons with HIV-related infections. Services for families and friends of persons with HIV-related infections were severely lacking (Smerke, 1988).

DENVER NURSING PROJECT IN HUMAN CARING

The Denver Nursing Project in Human Caring (DNPHC) was established through the collaborative efforts of one academic institution and two clinical agencies in July 1988. The DNPHC or Caring Center is a community-based, intergovernmentally sponsored, nurse-administered care center for Colorado residents with HIV-related infections and their significant others who are eligible to be or are already part of the DVAMC, DDHH, or UH systems. The three major goals of the Caring Center include:

1. Providing the clientele with choices, options, and meanings

2. Emphasizing optimal wellness and continuity of care

3. Not duplicating available services

The DNPHC Center is unique in many ways; it is the only nurse-administered care center for this clientele in the country, theoretically based on the philosophy of human caring, and intergovernmentally sponsored.

NEEDS ASSESSMENT

In the fall of 1987 nursing administrators of two clinical agencies (DVAMC and DDHH) identified deficits in continuity of care and gaps in services for HIV-positive and AIDS clients and their families. These deficits were not only detrimental to the well-being of the clients but also inefficient and costly. For example, some clients remained in the hospital far longer than medically indicated because supervised living arrangements were unavailable. Clients requiring an intravenous medication infusion or blood transfusion often were admitted to the hospital or to the emergency room when these procedures could have been done in an outpatient center. Demand for education and counseling of clients, families, and significant others had exceeded available resources.

Recognizing that neither agency could independently support a program to address these needs, the chief nursing executives of the two agencies explored the possibility of intergovernmental management. Current trends suggest that future forms of intergovernmental relations will look less like the traditional vertical relationships (federal to state to local) of previous decades, but rather will feature a series of agreements among various levels of governments. Cooperation among caregivers in diverse settings has been advocated as a key strategy in the response to the HIV epidemic (Koop, 1987).

A joint task force consisting of nurse clinicians and educators from

DVAMC and DDHH involved in the care of clients with HIV-related infections was formed to plan an integrated intergovernmental response to the two nursing services. Initially, the task force examined the phases of HIV infection, identified the client and family needs manifest in each phase, and detailed the requisite nursing care.

HIV INFECTION—CONTINUUM OF CARE

The five phases identified were: initiation, asymptomatic, early symptomatic, acute, and terminal (see Table 1). The first phase examined was initiation. The process for the client was being informed of the presence of the HIV infection. His/her needs could include grief, denial, and anger. Possible nursing care required included: returning control to patient, continuing activities, financial counseling, and assessing abilities to recognize and manage the following responsibilities: (1) *for others*: how to tell contacts and sex education; (2) *for outcome*: nutrition, hygiene, rest, and avoidance of reinfection; and (3) *assess patient and family needs*: knowledge of disease, need to see a physician, contact persons, and continuity of care.

The task force then identified three areas where adequate services were then available but heavily utilized: at the time of initial testing, during acute episodes requiring hospitalization, and hospice care. Deficits in services for both clients and their families during the early and intermediate phases of the infection were considerable. Further, available services were fragmented. In spite of the fact that HIV-related infections were generally accompanied by limited stamina, available physical, educational, and emotional support services had to be accessed from a variety of agencies and locations. In addition to the clients' and their families' experience of a physical burden posed by this lack of continuity, there was the added confusion of multiple relationships with care providers.

Clearly, persons with HIV-related infections and their families experience many unique and special needs requiring health professionals to recognize and deliver care compassionately and competently. Therefore, the task force sought consultation from the Center for Human Caring at the University of Colorado Health Sciences School of Nursing on the adoption of the philosophy and science of human caring as articulated by Watson (1979, 1985) as the theoretical framework for the project. As a result of this consultation, the three agencies formed the Denver Nursing Project in Human Caring (DNPHC) to provide community-based nursing services to persons with HIV-related infections and their significant others.

DNPHC CENTER'S PHILOSOPHY

The DNPHC Center is based on the philosophy and science of human caring. Historically, physical and psychological caring have been accepted as an integral component of nursing. Recently, clinicians, educators, and researchers in nursing have renewed their commitment to human caring, a compassion and concern for the client's total well-being as the essence of nursing. The needs of persons with HIV-related infections for physical and psychoemotional caring are paramount. The task force recommended a community-based nurse-administered care center providing education, physical, and support services within a caring milieu that emphasizes choice, optimal wellness, meaning, continuity of care, and maximal independence. That is, instead of focusing on the terminal nature of the disease, DNPHC Center would emphasize optimal well-being within a human caring theoretical framework for clients with HIV-related infections and their significant others. Recent research studies have elucidated human caring as the modality through which nurses facilitated the client's well-being and physical comfort (Benner, 1984; Brown, 1982, 1986; Condon, 1987; Gaut, 1984; Glick, 1986; Hester & Barcus, 1986; Larson, 1981, 1987; Mayer, 1986, 1987; Ray, 1984, 1987; Riemen, 1984; Sherwood, 1988; Swanson-Kauffman, 1986).

The philosophy and science of human caring has been grounded by Smerke (1988) within an interdisciplinary framework. Nine disciplines were selected to participate in the identification of the exemplary human caring literature. The disciplines selected included: psychoneuroimmunology, socio-behavioral sciences, anthropology, fine arts, philosophy, including ethics and humanities, theology, and nursing. From the hermeneutical analysis, seven major themes for the meanings of human caring emerged: genuine dialogue, authentic relationships/ encounters, understanding and respecting the essence of persons, complementary modality of healing, experiential process, making decisions/choices/judgments, and providing human/economic resource exchanges. The nurse and the client with HIV-related infections experience genuine dialogue during the caring interaction. Through dialogue, affirmation and acceptance of the other person occurs (Buber, 1965). Dialogue transmits human warmth, self-expression, gives courage to face problems, and awakens in him/her spiritual forces which give structure, life, and unity to him/her as a person (Tournier, 1987).

Clients who perceive that they are not being cared for experience a feeling of being less than a person; they feel like an object (Watson, 1985). Buber (1965) stated that the most beneficial relationship is when both persons are treated and respected as persons, not as objects. When persons experience caring, feelings of well-being are believed to ensue. In turn, these feelings can affect bodily processes and functions.

Caring means understanding and respecting the essence of the person. When the client experiences a caring interaction, the client perceives that he/she is being recognized by the nurse as a unique, thinking, and feeling human being. Caring promotes the respect and dignity of the person. Van Kaam (1959) stated that a seriously ill person experiences a narrower and changing world which becomes a lonely place. The ill client feels as an outsider in his/her once familiar world and he/she feels as a stranger in the life he/she has lived. When a nurse interacts with the client in a caring way, the established relationship will relieve the client of the loneliness of the illness world. Watson (1985) held that when clients experience caring, they have the capacity for self-healing. Healing enhances, promotes, and preserves the person (Pilisuk & Parks, 1986).

Caring is an experiential process. Watson's theory of human caring provides the nurse with 10 "carative" factors to guide his/her practice. Experiencing the caring between the client with HIV-related infections and the nurse, inner power and strength are released within the client, providing a broader perspective of the meaning of the situation. Inner harmony and self-healing processes are initiated. Through the caring transaction, the nurse and client experience self-knowledge, self-reverence, self-healing, and self-care processes. Self-control, choice, and self-determination within health-illness decisions are promoted by the nurse within the client-nurse relationship (Watson, 1985).

During the caring interaction, the nurse facilitates the making of decisions, choices, and judgments with the client. In allowing the client to make the choices and decisions, the nurse understands the client at face value and trusts the client.

Caring means providing human/economic resource exchanges for persons with HIV-related infections. Therefore, nurses play a major role in helping the client to gain inner strength, power, and self-healing through the caring transaction(s) (Watson, 1985).

Watson's philosophy and theory of the science of caring provides the DNPHC Center with a framework for delivering individually focused nursing care to persons with HIV-related infections. Watson defined caring as the moral ideal of nursing with "concern for preservation of humanity, dignity, and fullness of self" (1985, p. 14). In Watson's (1985) theory, the caring relationship is composed of three elements: the phenomenal field, the actual caring occasion, and transpersonal caring. The phenomenal field is the life space, or the totality of the experience and the individual's frame of reference. The actual caring occasion is an event and has a field greater than the occasion itself. The transpersonal caring transaction is an intersubjective human-to-human relationship. The caring transactions promote congruence between the perceptions and experiences of the person and promote self as is and ideal self, and harmony within the body-mind-spirit gestalt of the person. Through the caring transaction, inner power and strength are released. This helps the person gain a sense of inner harmony, self-healing processes are potentiated, and the meaning in the experience is found.

In Watson's (1985) theory, the client is the agent of the change. The nurse, however, can be a co-participant in the change process through the caring transaction. The nurse is not the agent of change; rather, the client's personal, internal, mental-spiritual mechanisms allow the self to be healed through various internal or external agents.

The nurse's role is one of facilitation. The nurse helps the client gain a higher degree of harmony within the mind, body, and soul which generates self-knowledge, self-reverence, self-healing, and self-care processes. The human-to-human caring transactions respond to the subjective inner world of the person, so that the nurse helps the client find meaning in his/her existence, disharmony, suffering, and/or turmoil and promotes self-control, choice, and self-determination with the health-illness decisions (Watson, 1985). The client gains capacity for self-healing, self-care, and enhanced well-being (Watson, 1985).

The relationship of psychoemotional and physical well-being is particularly relevant in immunologic diseases such as HIV-related infections. Negative emotions such as depression and anxiety can impede immune function and healing, whereas positive emotions such as hope can enhance healing (Locke & Colligan, 1986). Long-term survivors of AIDS have endorsed the importance of a positive state of mind in maintaining physical and psychoemotional well-being (Accola, 1988), but persons with AIDS-related illnesses experience many psychoemotional stressors which can cause negative emotions, such as alienation and expendability (Cohen & Weissman, 1986) and decreased self-esteem (Turner & Williamson, 1986).

The focus of nursing interventions within this theory is the caring transaction. The four intended consequences of the caring transactions are: (1) releasing of inner power and strength, generating and potentiating self-healing processes and finding meaning in the experience; (2) increasing the degree of transpersonal caring by increasing the degree of genuineness and sincerity of the nurse; (3) contributing to the person's developing spiritual essence or real self, and contributing to more self-knowledge, self-reverence, self-control, and self-healing for both nurse and client; and (4) creating a spiritual union between the two persons, where both are capable of transcending self, time, and space (Watson, 1985).

Watson's carative factors provide the nurse with theoretically-based caring strategies to guide his/her practice. Watson held that 7 of the 10 carative factors describe what the nurse does to provide care. These seven carative factors (Watson, 1985, p. 75) include:

1. Instillation of faith-hope

2. Development of a helping-trusting, human care relationship

3. Promotion and acceptance of the expression of positive and negative feelings

4. Creative problem-solving caring process

5. Promotion of transpersonal teaching-learning

6. Provision of a supportive, protective, and/or corrective mental, physical, sociocultural and spiritual environment

7. Assistance with the gratification of human needs

The remaining three carative factors describe the necessary qualities of the nurse. These three carative factors (Watson, 1985, p. 78) include:

1. Formation of a humanistic-altruistic system of values

2. Cultivation of sensitivity to self and others

3. Allowance for existential-phenomenological-spiritual forces

Drawing from Watson's work, it might be hypothesized that through the caring philosophy, value, and process, the client experiences inner power and strength and is able to transcend the present situation. The client is able to cope more effectively with the disease and enhance his/her level of well-being and physical comfort. The result will be a reintegration of the mind-body-spirit, which is the goal of nursing and well-being, even in the midst of pain, suffering, and diseases.

IMPLEMENTATION—THE FIRST NINE MONTHS

While there are many agencies that provide aspects of care for people with AIDS in the Denver metropolitan area, there is currently no single agency which provides the range of integrated, whole person nursing services provided by this project, not only for persons with AIDS but also for persons with an HIV-positive status and their significant others. Thus the DNPHC has responded to a significant unmet need in this community.

The DNPHC Center is housed in a free-standing building on the campus of DVAMC. No rent is currently being charged by DVAMC in lieu of services provided to the DVAMC clients, their families, and significant others. The building has 2,341 square feet, consisting of a treatment room, a day-activity room, two private offices for counseling and interviews, a secretary's office, a support group room, an educational room, a small space for the staff, storage area, and a public bathroom. Within the building are numerous paintings, flowers, a picture of the NAMES quilt, and plants. The physical environment is nonclinical and homelike even though technical and therapeutic measures are provided.

ORGANIZATIONAL STRUCTURE

A contractual agreement concerning the administration and management of the DNPHC Center has been established between the four agencies, DVAMC, DDHH, UCHSC - School of Nursing, and UH, including shared provision of staff and procedures for provision and payment for services and supplies. Clientele for the DNPHC are clients who are eligible or are being followed at DVAMC, DDHH, or UH. Since the DNPHC is a nurse-administered center, the medical care responsibility and accountability are retained by the client's primary physician. Referrals to the DNPHC Center, however, can be made by nurses, physicians, other clinical and community agencies, clients, significant others, or self. When the client enrolls at the DNPHC, an initial intake is done to ascertain the client's eligibility. The client's eligibility for services at DNPHC is verified by the nurse with the appropriate medical facility. If the client is being followed at one of the above facilities, he/she is eligible for services and his/her enrollment process is finalized.

The faculty associate, a .5 FTE position, is contributed by the University of Colorado Center for Human Caring, DVAMC, and DDHH. The faculty associate serves as the project director and promotes the integration of the philosophy and science of human caring with the staff, clients, and families; directs research; networks within the community; preceptors students; and oversees the entire project. The nursing care in the DNPHC Center is supervised by a Clinical Director (.5 FTE) contributed by the DVAMC and provided by registered nurses (one of whom has his PhD and 3 of whom are baccalaureate prepared for a 1.3 FTE total), two contributed by DDHH, one by DVAMC, and one by UH.

Personnel assigned to DNPHC Center have participated in an intensive 1-week philosophical, theoretical, and context orientation upon joining the staff. The on-going intensive educational experiences in the philosophical base and requisite physical and psychoemotional skills for caring with clients with HIV-related infections and their significant others provide the staff with an evolving framework for caring with this group of persons.

In addition to these formal positions, there is a cadre of professional volunteers, including psychiatric clinical nurse specialists and psychiatrists who conduct group sessions and individual therapy. Also, nonprofessional volunteers (clients, family members, lovers, and others) assume a variety of responsibilities, including clerical duties, cleaning, advertising, socialization, and fund raising. Many of the center's activities would not be possible without the support and contribution of these volunteers. Many of these volunteers are persons in early stages of the illness for whom volunteerism provides therapeutic activity through meaningful work in helping others.

Five committees were developed and initiated in order to facilitate the demanding needs of the center. Both staff and clients serve on the committees. A finance committee oversees the management of the donations and will conduct an initial assessment of the feasibility and process of third-party reimbursement. A fund raising committee coordinates the free Friday lunches, sends thank yous, and initiates benefits for the center. The volunteer committee is establishing the initial roles and responsibilities as well as a training program for the volunteers. The education and activity committee creates a monthly calender of all the activities and events planned by the center, publicizes the events, and oversees the clients' bimonthly newsletter. Finally, the policy and forms committee updates the policies and medication protocols and checks the crash cart.

POPULATION BEING SERVED

The DNPHC Center serves Colorado residents with HIV-related infections, their families, and significant others who are eligible to be or are already part of the DVAMC, DDHH, or UH systems. Responding to the demands for services imposed by the existing caseload of such clients, the DNPHC personnel secured interagency and community financial support and cooperation to open the DNPHC Center on a limited basis. The DNPHC Center has thus been in operation since July 25, 1988. The DNPHC Center is currently open only from 10:00 a.m. to 2 p.m., Monday through Thursday; 8:00 a.m. to 2 p.m. on Friday; and 6:30 p.m. to 8:30 p.m. on Tuesday and Thursday.

SERVICES CURRENTLY PROVIDED

Current services offered are limited due to personnel, time, and resources constraints. The services include symptom management, outpatient medical support, counseling and support, health promotion and education, and coordination and referral.

Symptom Management

Nursing management of the person with HIV-related infections includes assessment for common symptoms such as: pain; fatigue; fever, chills, and night sweats; weight loss; swollen lymph glands; pink, purple, or brown spots on skin; thrush or candida in mouth; persistent diarrhea; dry cough; memory deficits; and loss of balance. Assessment is followed by appropriate nursing intervention and referral where indicated. Nursing interventions include traditional approaches, such as skin care, client teaching related to pain management and energy conservation, and recognition and management of physical crisis. In addition one or more of the following complementary caring modalities are available to the client and significant others: relaxation therapy, meditation, massage therapy, therapeutic touch, and guided imagery/ visualization.

Outpatient Medical Support

The needs of clients with HIV-related infections require medical interventions at times. The medical support available includes the administration of IV medication therapy (Amphotericin, pentamidine, fluids), blood transfusions, nebulized pentamidine, education about medication, and monitoring the client's compliance and any adverse effects.

Counseling and Support

Persons with HIV-related infections and their significant others have a great need for counseling and support. The DNPHC Center provides the following services: individual client counseling, family/significant others counseling and support, stress management, support groups (two open groups are available for homosexuals, family members, lovers, IV drug abusers, and others), and memories (a monthly evening for closure, a time to remember those who have died from the virus). A buddy system (friendship and a home care program) is still being formulated.

Health Promotion and Education

A variety of health promotion and disease prevention strategies are utilized within the DNPHC. First, the lack of knowledge among the newly diagnosed clients with HIV-related infections and their families is a critical problem. Therefore individual and group educational opportunities are provided and include content on: the immunology of AIDS, HIV testing, transmission and prevention of the spread of the virus, sex education, caring for HIV-positive people at home, specific opportunistic infections, and other related diseases. All new staff participate in an orientation program that includes information on the teaching of clients. All staff nurses also participate in the educational component of the project. In addition, the staff have provided educational classes to other nursing units within the hospital, industries, and community groups.

Second, classes are available to volunteers (usually HIV-positive themselves), clients, and their significant others in the implementation of complementary caring modalities. The educational program prepares these participants to use such strategies as therapeutic touch, relaxation, and simple guided imagery with themselves or with the persons for whom they are caring. This activity is viewed as an innovative and empowering approach to health promotion in this population. Rather than being reduced to a position of despair, hopelessness, and helplessness, the provider of these healing strategies is empowered through caring. This empowerment in itself may be a powerful tool for healing, that is, for finding meaning, purpose, and peace in one's life regardless of the length of that life. In addition, a growing body of literature suggests that positive emotions (such as love and caring) may impact on the immune system in a positive way (Borysenko, 1985; Dillon, Minchoff & Baker, 1985-1986) and may be a powerful approach to health promotion.

Third, wellness classes are developed and offered to cover such areas as nutrition, modified exercise, and intimacy/relationships. Finally, classes related to loss and death and dying are developed for persons with HIV-related infections and their families. Content in these classes includes not only the psycho-social-spiritual aspects of death and dying but also the pragmatic aspects with which each dying person and his/her significant others must deal.

Coordination and Referral

The staff and volunteers work closely with health care professionals and community advocacy groups to coordinate care. An integral component of the DNPHC Center is the promotion and facilitation of the relationship of the client with the physician providing the medical care. Physicians, as well as nurses, social workers, psychiatrists, and nutritionists are also invited to work with their clients as required in the DNPHC Center rather than in the acute care setting.

The demands which the person with AIDS faces are multifaceted and involve multiple levels of the health care and social systems. At a time when energy is waning, these persons frequently find themselves in the position of having to negotiate more and more fragments of the social system. Housing, transportation, employment, obtaining benefits, and the like are all areas with which the AIDS client and significant others must deal.

SERVICES FOR STAFF

In addition to the services available for the clientele, services are provided by the DNPHC to the staff. They include: allocated time for daily group centering (a method of empowerment for the staff and a form of healing and wholeness for the center, a time to become genuinely present with those around them and focused on the current activities), bimonthly support groups (the promotion of empowerment and healing within the staff and a time to share one's own feelings), and staff meetings (to keep abreast of current research findings and administrative needs of the center and sponsoring agencies). When working with this clientele, there is a great need for the staff to experience caring with self and caring with others in order to decrease the amount of anxiety, grief, frustration, and burnout.

EXAMPLE OF A DAY AT THE DNPHC

When a new client comes to the center for the first visit, he or she signs the patient log, records name, social security number, and agency; notes if this is his or her first visit; and in which activities he or she wishes to participate. Currently there are 80 different activities that have been assigned a code number for statistical purposes. There is always flexibility for additional services to be made available as the need arises. The client is given a tour of the center. In addition, the available services and activities are explained. Then a complete intake is done with a nurse.

The intake incorporates the six major services offered by the center. The client's symptoms are assessed and recorded. The client's current medical support is elicited and his/her support systems are assessed. The knowledge level of the client is assessed and information is provided when appropriate. Finally, the client's financial, housing, and spiritual concerns are discussed and evaluated. The nurse then becomes the case manager for this client. Together, the nurse and the client complete a care plan. A summary is recorded from the initial intake. Mutual goals are established between the client and the nurse. Any protocols the client is involved in are recorded. Finally, the carative factors being implemented with the corresponding interventions are documented on an on-going basis.

DOCUMENTATION

A separate chart is kept on each client utilizing the center. The chart includes a care plan, progress notes, intake form, list of available services, medical history and physical, and psychiatric history if applicable. All forms are color coded for easy reference. A modified SOAPE— subjective, objective, assessment, plan, and evaluation—format is utilized by all disciplines on the same progress notes. With every visit, a notation is made on the chart. The note begins with A (Assessment); P (Plan): Watson's carative factors are used for the plans which are theoretically based strategies; I (Interventions): how the carative factor(s) were carried out; and E (Evaluation). After the progress note is completed on both sides, it is photocopied; the original progress note is placed in the client's chart and the copy remains in the Center's chart.

PAYMENT POLICY

Currently, payment for DVAMC clients is handled through the routing slip mechanisms at the DVAMC. A routing slip is completed after each client visit to the DNPHC Center. The routing slip is then sent to Medical Administrative Services (MAS) for accounting purposes. Clients from the other agencies are theoretically billed directly by the agency for the services and supplies they received at the DNPHC Center. A copy of the log book is sent to each agency monthly with a list of their clients and their significant others, services utilized, and supplies used.

STATISTICS

During the first 11 months, the DNPHC Center has had 1,598 visits from 120 clients. The DNPHC Center has prevented 104 hospital days, shortened the hospital stay for 5 clients by at least 7 days each, and eliminated 72 IV medication administrations in the emergency room. The remarkable increase in visits in a very short amount of time serves as confirmation from clients that the DNPHC is fulfilling a need unmet elsewhere in the health care system. Also, to date, the DNPHC Center has increased access to nursing care and education for the target clientele and operates within a human caring framework which emphasizes optimal wellness, individual choices, meanings, and continuity of care for the clientele and their significant others.

One of the primary goals of starting the DNPHC was to provide more effective and cost efficient care for this clientele. The District AIDS Task Force Report (1988) prepared by Dr. R. Ellison and Linda Laxson, BSN, RN, CIC for the DVAMC demonstrates the sudden decrease in hospital admissions and inpatient hospital days from July to December 1988 even though the number of outpatient visits to the Infectious Disease Clinic increased. They held that this decrease was directly related to the increase in visits to the DNPHC for blood transfusions, IV medications, symptom management, and the other services (see Table 2).

RESEARCH BEING CONDUCTED

Three nursing research studies are currently being conducted at the DNPHC:

1. Assessing the implementation of the philosophy and theory of human caring in clinical practice. The client's record is the data. Each client's plan and interventions are transcribed onto the computer and subjected to a hermeneutical analysis. Hermeneutics means an analysis of text and is used to interpret and explain the carative factors. Exemplars of the carative factors are being generated from this clinical practice setting.

2. Discovery of the meanings of human caring from persons with HIV-related infections. Clients attending the center are being interviewed using nonstructured formats. The emerging themes and unity of meaning are being generated by a phenomenological inquiry.

3. Cost-effectiveness of nurse managed centers. Statistics are recorded monthly on the utilization of services by the clients and the estimated savings to the institutions.

CLIENTS' EXPERIENCES

For many of the clients, the DNPHC represents "my home." The center has become a "safe place" for them to go. In the Caring Center, the clients have experienced love, friendship, support, compassion, warmth, empathy, and caring. One client stated, "You can feel the caring around you. There's a real kind of loving, warm feeling that goes through your body and you can't pass by that nurse and not smile again. The staff is available to hug you and hold you and listen to you. You don't have to say anything." Another client stated, "It is a place I can go to talk with other people who have the same or similar problems." These are only a few of the many examples of the clients' experiences.

IMPACT ON NURSING

The DNPHC Center is innovative on several levels: as a model of intergovernmental management, a model of wellness-based compassionate caring, and a generalized economic model for the care of persons with AIDS and AIDS-related illnesses. In addition, the DNPHC not only addresses the imperatives from the Presidential Commission (1988) to implement new models of nurse-managed care for persons with AIDS and to emphasize noninstitutional care but also incorporates innovative approaches to the organization of the delivery of nursing care and development of autonomous nursing roles, both of which have been identified as important strategies to easing the growing shortage of nurses (Kramer & Schmalenberg, 1988; Mabbett, 1987; Sigma Theta Tau, 1987).

IMPACT OF THE DNPHC CARING CENTER ON THE COMMUNITY

The DNPHC Center has made a tremendous impact on the community. Many of the referrals received come from the clientele who are utilizing the services. The DNPHC Center has become known in the community. The community has supported the center with free lunches on Fridays. It is also receiving many inquires and referrals from different community agencies. The center has increased access to nursing care and education for the target clientele, has fulfilled an unmet need in the community, and has gained the community trust and support.

FUTURE TREND OF NURSE-MANAGED CARE CENTERS

The future trend in health care delivery systems for chronic and terminal illnesses will be nurse-administered care centers. People are not willing to give up their control to other people, including health care professionals. Nurse-managed centers provide terminally ill clients with empowerment and decision-making strategies for their own health/illness decisions. As nurses, we have the ability and creativity to develop and initiate innovative and autonomous roles, and creating nurse-managed centers will make a dramatic impact on the health care delivery system. We can provide not only efficient but also cost-effective care and an environment that promotes healing and wholeness for clients and their significant others.

REFERENCES

Accola, J. (1988, May 27). Pair claim AIDS cured: Men credit holistic medicine for the current good health. *Rocky Mountain News*.

Anderson, D. (1988). *The mountain—plains ETC: AIDS and the rural response*. Unpublished manuscript.

Benner, P. (1984). *From novice to expert*. Menlo Park, CA: Addison-Wesley.

Borysenko, J. (1985). Healing motives: An interview with David McClelland. *Advances, 2*(2), 29–41.

Brown, L. (1982). Behaviors of nurses perceived by hospitalized patients as indicators of care. *Dissertation Abstracts International, 42*(11), 4361-B. (University Microfilms No. DA 82-09, 803).

Brown, L. (1986). The experiences of care: Patient perspectives. *Topics in Clinical Nursing, 8*(2), 56–62.

Buber, M. (1965). *The knowledge of man: A philosophy of the interhuman*. New York: Harper & Row.

Centers for Disease Control (CDC). (1988). *AIDS weekly surveillance report—United States*. Atlanta; Georgia: Author, May 16.

Cohen, M.A., & Weissman, H.W. (1986). A biopsychosocial approach to AIDS. *Psychosomatics, 27*(4), 245–249.

Condon, E.H. (1987). *A phenomenological analysis of the experience of being caring in a nurse-client interaction*. Unpublished doctoral dissertation, The University of Texas at Austin.

Dillon, K.M., Minchoff, B., & Baker, K. (1985–86). Positive emotional states and enhancement of the immune system. *International Journal of Psychiatry in Medicine, 15*, 13–17.

District AIDS task force report. (1988). *Patient workload for HIV patients at Denver VAMC, October 1986 to December 1988*. Unpublished manuscript.

Droste, T. (1987). Going home to die: Developing home health services for AIDS patients. *Hospitals, 61*(16), 54–56.

Gaut, D.A. (1984). A theoretic description of caring as action. In M. Leininger (Ed.), *Care: The essence of nursing and health* (pp. 27–44). Thorofare, NJ: Slack.

Glick, M.S. (1986). Caring touch and anxiety in myocardial infarction patients in the intermediate cardiac care unit. *Intensive Care Nursing, 2*(2), 61–66.

Goff, W., & McDonough, P. (1986). A community health approach to AIDS: Caring for the patient educating the public. *Journal of Community Health Nursing, 3*(4), 191–200.

Hay, L. (1986). *You can heal your life*. Santa Monica, CA: Hay House.

Hay, L. (1988). *The AIDS book: Creating a positive approach*. Santa Monica, CA: Hay House.

Hester, N., & Barcus, C. (1986). *The human experience of pain for hospitalized children*. Unpublished manuscript.

HIV/AIDS monthly statistics. (1989). The Colorado Department of Health, May.

Institute of Medicine. (1988). *Confronting AIDS: Update 1988*. Washington, DC: National Academy Press.

Institute of Medicine and National Academy of Sciences. (1986). *Confronting AIDS*. Washington, DC: National Academy Press.

Koop, C.E. (1987). An AIDS health care network: The time is now. *AIDS Patient Care, 1*(1), 1–2.

Kramer, M., & Schmalenberg, C. (1988). Magnet hospitals; Part I. *Journal of Nursing Administration, 18*(1), 13–31.

Larson, P.J. (1981). Oncology patients' and professional nurses' perceptions of important nurse caring behaviors. *Dissertation Abstracts International, 42*(02), 568. (University Microfilms No. ADG81-16511).

Larson, P.J. (1987). Comparison of cancer patients' and professional nurses' perceptions of important nurse caring behaviors. *Heart and Lung, 16*(2), 187–193.

Locke, S., & Colligan, D. (1986). *The healer within: The new medicine of mind and body*. New York: New American Library.

Mabbett, P. (1987). From burned out to turned on to skills of personal energy management and "caring." *Canadian Nurse, 83*(3), 15–19.

Matthews-Simonton, S., Simonton, O., & Creighton, J. (1984). *Getting well again*. New York: Bantam Books.

Mayer, D.K. (1986). Cancer patients' and families' perceptions of nurse caring behaviors. *Topics in Clinical Nursing, 8*(2), 63–69.

Mayer, D.K. (1987). Oncology nurses' versus cancer patients' perceptions of nurses caring behaviors: A replication study. *Oncology Nursing Forum, 14*(3), 48–52.

McCaffrey, E. (1987). Setting up an AIDS unit: The Johns Hopkins' experience. *AIDS Patient Care, 1*(1), 6–8.

———. (1988). *Needs assessment of persons with HIV-related infections and their families at the DVAMC and DDHH*. Unpublished manuscript.

O'Brien, A.M., Oerlemans-Buan, M., & Blanchfield, J.C. (1987). Nursing the AIDS patient at home. *AIDS Patient Care, 1*(1), 21–24.

Pilisuk, M. & Parks, S.H. (1986). *The healing web: Social networks and human survival*. Hanover, NH: University Press of New England.

Presidential Commission on the Human Immunodeficiency Virus Epidemic. (1988). *Interim Report—March, 1988.* Washington, D.C.

Ray, M.A. (1984). The development of a classification system of institutional caring. In M. Leininger (Ed.), *Care: The essence of nursing and health* (pp. 95–112). Thorofare, NJ: Slack.

Ray, M.A. (1987). Technological caring: A new model in critical care. *Dimensions of Critical Care Nursing, 6*(3), 166–173.

Riemen, D.J. (1984). The essential structure of a caring interaction: A phenomenological study. *Dissertation Abstracts International, 44*(10), 3041.

Serinus, J. (1987). *Psychoimmunity & the healing process.* (2nd ed.) Berkeley, CA: Celestial Arts.

Sherwood, G. (1988). *Nurse's caring as perceived by post-operative patients: A phenomenological study.* Unpublished doctoral dissertation, The University of Texas at Austin.

Siegel, B. (1986). *Love, medicine, & miracles: Lessons learned about self-healing from a surgeon's experience with exceptional patients.* New York: Aslan Publishing.

Sigma Theta Tau. (1987). *Arista '87: Nurses and the delivery of Health Care Services* (Monograph). Indianapolis, IN.

Smerke, J. (1988). *Needs assessment of persons with HIV-related infections and their families at the DVAMC and DDHH.* Unpublished manuscript.

Smerke, J. (1988). *The discovery and creation of the meanings of human caring through the development of a guide to the caring literature.* Unpublished doctoral dissertation, The University of Colorado.

Smith, A.M. (1987). Alternatives in AIDS homecare. *AIDS Patient Care, 1*(1), 28–32.

Swanson-Kauffman, K.M. (1986). Caring in the instance of unexpected early pregnancy loss. *Topics in Clinical Nursing, 8*(2), 37–46.

Tournier, P. (1987). *A listening ear: Reflections on Christian caring.* Minneapolis: Augsburg Publishing.

Turner, J.G., & Williamson, K.M. (1986). AIDS: A challenge for contemporary nursing part II: Clinical AIDS. *Focus on Critical Care, 13*(4), 41–50.

Van Kaam, A. (1959). The nurse in the patient's world. *The American Journal of Nursing, 59*(12), 1708–1710.

Watson, J. (1979). *Nursing: The philosophy and science of caring.* Boston: Little, Brown.

Watson, J. (1985). *Nursing: Human science and human care. A theory of nursing.* Norwalk, CT: Appleton-Century-Crofts.

World Health Organization. (1989). *AIDS update*. Geneva: Author.

Worldwide number of AIDS/HIV cases up 40 percent. (1989). *The American Nurse, 21*(6), 7.

TABLE 1
HIV Infection Continuum of Care

Phase	Process	Nursing Care

Initiation	Informed
	HIV infected
	Grief: Denial and
	   anger
		Return control to client
		Continue activities
		Financial counseling
		Assess abilities to recognize and
		   manage responsibilities:
		  1. *For others*
		    a. How to tell contacts
		    b. Sex education
		  2. *For outcome*
		    a. Nutrition
		    b. Hygiene
		    c. Rest
		    d. Avoid reinfection
		  3. *Assess patient and family needs*
		    a. Knowledge of disease
		    b. Physician
		    c. Contact person
		    d. Continuity of care

Asymptomatic	Few physical
	   problems
	Self-worth questions
	Integrity vs.
	   despair
	Suicide
		Channel energies to help others and/
		   or make life meaningful
		Support group
		Wellness activities
		Direct to activities that may leave a
		   legacy
		Reinforcement

Early Symptomatic	Decreased energy
	   level
	Weight Loss
	Depression
	Respiratory infection
	Diarrhea
	Dementia
	Skin-pressure
	   sores/diarrhea
		Symptomatic support
		AZT therapy:
		  1. Compliance
		  2. Manage adverse effect
		    a. Bone marrow
		    b. Drug intox
		    c. Nausea and vomiting
		    d. Headache
		Housekeeper/homemaker support
		Supervision
		Energy conservation
		Nutrition

Acute	Infections	Hospitalized for work-up, but then outpatient
	Kaposi's sarcoma	Administer IV drugs:
	Neuropathies	1. Pentamidine
	Dementia	2. Chemotherapy
		3. Other drugs
		Transportation to clinic
		Physical care/comfort
		1. Pain management
		2. Supportive
		Choices: How to die (COR, ICU, antibiotics, blood)
		Respite for caregivers
Terminal	Systems failure	Referral to hospice
(average length	Suicide attempts	Reminiscence
of time: 2 years)		Continue care/comfort

TABLE 2

Patient Workload for HIV Patients at Denver VAMC, October 1986 to December 1988

	Hospital Admissions	Hospital Inpatient Days	Outpt Visits[1]	Outpt Visits, DNPHC[2]	Outpt Tx by DNPHC
Oct–Dec 1986	14	239	50		
Jan–Jun 1987	38	460	203		
July–Dec 1987	55	519	368		
Jan–Jun 1988	64	690	592		
Jul–Dec 1988	49	549	643	471	71

[1]Outpatient visits to Infectious Disease clinic are counted. Data does not include visits to other clinics or walk-in visits to emergency room but does include a small percentage of non-HIV-infected patients.
[2]DNPHC: Denver Nursing Project in Human Caring
SOURCE: *District AIDS Task Force Report* (1989).

8

A REVIEW OF THE STATE OF THE ART OF RESEARCH ON NURSING CENTERS

Susan K. Riesch, DNSc, RN, FAAN
Professor
University of Wisconsin–Milwaukee
School of Nursing
Milwaukee, Wisconsin

The purpose of this chapter is to review the research that has been conducted on or in nursing centers to make recommendations for the future. The emphasis is upon the results of the studies. Readers are referred to the extensive bibliography to analyze further the literature.

OVERVIEW

Early nursing centers were developed to provide service. Since the 1970s, nursing centers have developed to include an additional potential as research and learning environments. Systematic investigations have determined the location of such centers and established a consensus definition, documented the issues of implementation, and explored student and patient/clinic outcomes. Conceptualization and organization of nursing centers have been diverse, including traditional public health, visiting nurse, community health, and institutional outreach models; wellness and health promotion models; and faculty practice and nurse entrepreneur models. This review is limited to the first two models, however.

LOCATION

Boettcher (1986) conducted a telephone survey to identify academic based centers in order to use them as a sample for her doctoral dissertation. Barger (1986b) surveyed all National League for Nursing (NLN)-accredited baccalaureate and master's programs and located 51 centers. With the establishment of an NLN Council for Nursing Centers, the locations can be monitored more readily.

Definition

The literature contains a number of definitions of nursing centers. Since the 1970s, the most common thread among the published definitions is that of direct access to nurses by clients. In 1984, a Delphi survey was conducted with a sample of 143 nurses attending the Second Biennial Conference on Nursing Centers. The Delphi questionnaire was developed by Fehring, Schulte, and Riesch (1987) to reflect the chief issues found in the literature. The following frequently quoted definition resulted:

> Nursing centers are organizations that provide direct access to professional nurses who offer holistic client-centered health services for reimbursement. With the use of nursing models of health, professional nurses in nursing centers diagnose and treat human responses to potential and actual health problems. Examples of professional nursing services include health education, health promotion, and health-related research. Services are targeted to individuals and groups whose health needs are not being met (e.g., the poor, women, elderly, minorities). An effective referral system and collaboration with other health care professionals are an integral part of nursing centers. As models of professional nursing practice and research, nurse-managed centers are ideal sites for faculty and student practice. They are administered by a professional nurse. (p. 62)

ISSUES OF IMPLEMENTATION

Much of the literature on the issues of implementation is anecdotal in nature with authors sharing their experiences. However, valuable knowledge is gained from a perusal of this literature. Barger (1986a) succinctly identified the issues as: (a) selection of clientele, (b) scope of practice, (c) physical facilities, (d) marketing, (e) personnel, (f) role of students, (g) financial base, (h) quality assurance and productivity, and (i) research and development. These issues are addressed in a monograph published by the American Nurses' Association (Aydelotte et al., 1987).

OUTCOMES OF HOSPITAL BASED NURSE RUN INSTITUTIONAL OUTREACH CLINICS

Nurse-run institutional outreach clinics were established in the late 1960s or early 1970s chiefly to develop an efficient care system for outpatients. Lewis and Resnick (1967) demonstrated increased satisfaction among patients with nurse-managed care; fewer incidents of seeking medical attention for minor complaints; decreased missed appointment rates from 10% to 5%; fewer hospital days, from 34.2 days/1000 patients in the nurse clinic compared with 126.1 days/1000 patients in the physician clinic; and shorter hospital stays when patients were hospitalized than was documented in the physician-run clinic.

In 1973, Allison showed that patients cared for in a nurse-run clinic had increased control of their blood sugar levels, improved healing of leg ulcers and infections, reduced hospital admissions, and decreased no-show rate (from 35% to 9%) when compared with their prior experience in the physician-run clinic. Hill (1986) documented, in England, that rheumatology outpatients reported greater satisfaction with their care and more personal attention in the nursing clinic compared with whatever clinic they had received care in previously.

OUTCOMES OF COMMUNITY HEALTH, WELLNESS, AND HEALTH PROMOTION CLINICS

Several nursing center leaders have taken their practice to the community and have demonstrated significant outcomes. Begun as a 1-month trial project, but still in existence today, is the Pine Street Inn. An innovation between the Boston Department of Health and Hospitals and Boston City Hospital, the Inn serves the homeless. Based on many years of documentation with the Inn's guests, Lenehan, McInnis, O'Donnell, and Hennessey (1985) demonstrated reduced emergency room visits, standardized nursing care plans for common health status alterations, and numerous individual case study successes such as a peaceful death or a family reuniting after a death.

Jameison and Martinson (1988) reported that, as a result of their Neighborhood Nurse program, 85% of their clients would have been hospitalized. Further, the cost of providing the program was 24% less than the minimum cost of a nursing home. Family involvement in the care of the elderly relative also was increased for clients in the program.

The most sophisticated and in-depth evaluation of patient/client outcomes was conducted by Kos and Rothberg (1981). The Adelphi University and Molloy College of Nursing collaborated to develop the Nursing Center for Family Health Services which functioned from 1972 to 1977 in the Moxby Ridge Apartments in New York. The patient/clinic outcomes consisted of changes in health knowledge, attitudes, and behavior; satisfaction with the care; and quality and cost-effectiveness of the care. Data were collected in three ways: using paper and pencil instruments, interviews, and external review by the Albert Einstein College of Medicine Department of Community Health. Outcomes included: (a) health perceptions that were future oriented; (b) appropriate use of medical resources based on self-evaluation of symptoms; (c) immunization compliance of 83%; (d) above average ratings on preventive, maternity, and pediatric care; (e) average cost-effectiveness: $42 per visit compared with a range in the geographic area of $37.50 to $50; and (f) low utilization: 1.8 staff seeing 5.5 patients per day. The report would have been enhanced if the instrumentation had been better described.

This clinic closed. The authors offered poor transportation, isolated location, a too small patient pool, and unresponsive reimbursement system as the reasons. They offer extensive advice to persons attempting to develop and maintain a nursing clinic.

Another study coming out of the Nursing Center for Family Health was Jones' (1976) documentation of health problems as they occur along the lifespan. Based on over 400 clients from birth through old age, Jones also made significant recommendations for the prevention of these health problems and/or their treatment. These findings could be incorporated into protocols for nursing center clients.

Nurses of the Louisville Visiting Nurses' Association began a Preventive Health Program (PHP) to serve persons over 65 through 20 clinics in the areas of health assessment, screening, education, and referral. To evaluate their first goal of early detection of disease, Newman, Sloss, and Anderson (1984) evaluated the number of persons screened over a 2-year period, the percent found to have a positive test, and the percent with a confirmed diagnosis after being referred. These data were compared with national and state data to calculate expected positives. The PHP outcome data were judged to be in line with outcomes from similar screening programs.

The second goal was the prevention of health problems and complications from existing chronic conditions. The unit of analysis was number of annual physician visits by clients. An earlier study in the Louisville area revealed that noninstitutionalized older adults visited their physician an average of 4.4 times per year and 25% made no physician visit. The PHP sample made 3.3 visits annually with 4% making no visit at all. Newman et al. (1984) presented an excellent idea and compared their own data with that of national, state, and local data sets.

Nichols (1985a & 1985b) conducted extensive analyses of the patients and families of the Yale Nurse Midwifery Service. She was able to describe her clients and compare her demographics and birthing outcomes with other nurse midwifery services. Additionally, she evaluated her postdate and postmature pregnancies and births and developed a protocol for their care. This is a significant contribution to the practice of nurse midwifery and an excellent example of the type of research that can be conducted in a nurse-controlled practice setting.

Many centers offer information and support groups for persons and families coping with a disease or undergoing a significant life event. Two studies address the outcomes of these groups. First, Duffy and Halloran (1987) developed and evaluated an information and support group for parents of children with asthma. They developed instruments to measure parents' knowledge and perceptions of their children's asthma and their understanding and ability to deal with the asthma. After participation in the group, parents reported improvements in their knowledge, perceptions, understanding, and ability to deal with the asthma. Not only did these nurses demonstrate effective, cost-efficient (group teaching being less costly than individual teaching) care, they developed valid research measures. Both the program and the instruments should be used by others.

In another study, expectant mothers and their coaches were found to have an increased perception of self-care after participation in childbirth preparation classes (Riesch, 1988). Many additional recommendations for study resulted from this analysis.

A frequently cited outcome is client satisfaction. Based on studies by Riesch (1985), Bagwell (1987), and Greshem-Kenton and Wisby (1987), it can be said that nursing center clients are well satisfied with the care. These investigations have contributed to the definition criteria that should be included in a comprehensive evaluation of client satisfaction.

STUDENT OUTCOMES

Though many authors state that student learning is one of the goals of their center, only one study was located that documented student outcomes. Hauf (1977) compared senior community health nursing students at the Montana State University on five measures to determine if they could meet the community health learning objectives to the same extent at the Nursing Center site as they could in the traditional public health site. She found no differences among the students except that students in the nursing center site spent less time orienting to the facility and more time in interaction with patients and their families than the traditional site students.

CONCLUSIONS AND RECOMMENDATIONS

Based on the studies reviewed there is no question that nursing center clients are satisfied and that nursing center leaders have contributed to the definition of independent, cost-effective practice. The research, however, is chiefly atheoretical, using small sample sizes and often obscure instruments, lacking control conditions, and not replicated. Further, nursing centers are not in the mainstream of health care delivery and are woefully underutilized and underfunded.

Therefore, it seems timely that a large multisite study be conducted to: (a) evaluate the scientific adequacy of the many protocols for care, (b) document the outcomes of care, and (c) develop a standardized method of data collection and analysis for client and clinic data, quality of care, and cost of care. No qualitative studies were located; thus, the experiences of nursing center clients from their perspective remains a fertile area for research. Nursing centers are ideal sites for pilot studies, instrument development, nursing diagnosis validation studies (Fehring & Frenn, 1986), and protocol evaluation.

Thus, as research environments (as well as practice and learning environments), nursing centers are underutilized. As Barger (1987) stated, nursing centers have potential for the conduct of research using Bloch's (1985) five categories of research: fundamentals of nursing care, nursing practice, nursing professional issues, delivery of nursing care, and nursing education. Further, if data are collected carefully, they can be compared with existing local, state, and national databases.

In summary, it has been my experience that nurses involved in nursing centers are among the warmest, least arrogant, and most creative people I've had the pleasure of working with. They are attempting to provide a type of care that many patients/clients and their families need and desire. Perhaps we could use all the excellent outcomes documented to date to catapult us into the mainstream of health care delivery.

REFERENCES

Adyelotte, M.K., Barger, S.E., Branstetter, E., Fehring, R.J., Lindgren, K., Lundeen, S., McDaniel, S., & Riesch, S.K. (1987). *The nursing center: Concept and design.* (Available from the American Nurses' Association, 2420 Pershing Road, Kansas City, MO 64108.)

Allison, S.E. (1973). A framework for nursing action in a nurse-conducted diabetic management clinic. *Journal of Nursing Administration, 3,* 53–60.

Bagwell, M.A. (1987). Client satisfaction with nursing center services. *Journal of Community Health Nursing, 4,* 29–42.

Barger, S.E. (1986a). Academic nurse-managed centers: Issues of implementation. *Family and Community Health, 9*, 12–22.

Barger, S.E. (1986b). Academic nursing centers: A demographic profile. *Journal of Professional Nursing, 2*, 246–251.

Barger, S.E. (1987). The potential for resources and research use in academic nurse managed centers. *Nurse Educator, 12*, 19–22.

Bloch, D.A. (1985). A conceptualization of nursing research and nursing science. In J.C. McCloskey & H.G. Grace (Eds.), *Current issues in nursing (*2nd ed.*)* (pp. 130–143). Boston: Blackwell Scientific.

Boettcher, J.M.H. (1986). *A national overview of nurse-managed centers.* Paper presented at the meeting of the Third Biennial Conference on Nursing Centers, Scottsdale, AZ.

Duffy, D., & Halloran, M.C. (1987). Effect of an educational program on parents of children with asthma. *Childrens' Health Care, 16*, 76–81.

Fehring, R.J., Schulte, J.A., & Riesch, S.K. (1986). Toward a definition of nurse-managed centers. *Journal of Community Health Nursing, 3*, 59–67.

Fehring, R.J., & Frenn, M. (1986). Nursing diagnosis in a nurse-managed wellness resource center. In M.F. Hurley (Ed.), *Classification of nursing diagnosis: Proceedings of the sixth conference* (pp. 401–407). St. Louis: Mosby.

Greshem-Kenton, L., & Wisby, M. (1987). Development and implementation of nurse-managed health program: A problem-oriented approach. *Journal of Ambulatory Care Management, 10*, 20–29.

Hauf, B.J. (1977). An evaluative study of a nursing center for community health nursing student experiences. *Journal of Nursing Education, 16*, 7–11.

Hill, J. (1986). Patient evaluation of a rheumatology nursing clinic. *Nursing Times, 82*(27), 42–43.

Jameison, M., & Martinson, I. (1988). *The Block Nurse Program: Neighbors helping neighbors.* Paper presented at the meeting of the Fourth Biennial Conference on Nursing Centers, Milwaukee, WI.

Jones, A. (1976). Overview of a nursing center for family health services in Freeport. *Nurse Practitioner, 1*, 26–31.

Kos, B.A., & Rothberg, J.S. (1981). Evaluation of a freestanding nurse clinic. In L.H. Aiken (Ed.), *Health policy and nursing practice* (pp. 19–42). New York: McGraw-Hill.

Lenehan, G.P., McInnis, B.N., O'Donnell, D., & Hennessey, M. (1985). A nurses' clinic for the homeless. *American Journal of Nursing, 85*, 1237–1240.

Lewis, E.E., & Resnick, B.A. (1967). Nurse clinics and progressive ambulatory patient care. *New England Journal of Medicine, 277,* 1236–1241.

Newman, J., Sloss, G.S., & Anderson, S. (1984). Evaluation of a health program. *Geriatric Nursing, 5,* 234–238.

Nichols, C.W. (1985a). The Yale Nurse Midwifery practice: Addressing the outcomes. *Journal of Nurse-Midwifery, 30,* 159–165.

Nichols, C.W. (1985b). Postdate pregnancy: Part II clinical implications. *Journal of Nurse-Midwifery, 30,* 259–268.

Riesch, S.K. (1988). Changes in the exercise of self-care agency: The childbearing dyad. *Western Journal of Nursing Research, 10,* 257–266.

Riesch, S.K. (1985). A primary care initiative: Nurse-managed centers. In M.D. Mezey & D.O. McGivern (Eds.), *Nurses, Nurse Practitioners* (pp. 242–248). Boston: Little, Brown.

BIBLIOGRAPHY

Adylotte, M.K., Barger, S.E., Branstetter, E., Fehring, R.J., Lindgren, K., Lundeen, S., McDaniel, S., & Riesch, S.K. (1987). *The nursing center: Concept and design.* (Available from the American Nurses' Association, 2420 Pershing Rd., Kansas City, MO 64108.)

Adylotte, M.K., Hardy, M.A., & Hope, K.L. (1988). *Nurses in private practice.* (Available from the American Nurses' Association, 2420 Pershing Rd., Kansas City, MO 64108.)

Allison, S.E. (1973). A framework for nursing action in a nurse-conducted diabetic management clinic. *Journal of Nursing Administration, 3,* 53–60.

Androwich, I., Hackbarth, D., & Swanson, L. (1984). *Collaborative nursing service: Nursing education model of a university medical center based community nursing service.* Paper presented at the Second Biennial Conference on Nurse Managed Centers, Milwaukee, WI.

Arlton, D.M., & Miercort, O.S. (1980). A nursing clinic: The challenge for student learning opportunities. *Journal of Nursing Education, 19,* 53–58.

Bagwell, M.A. (1987). Client satisfaction with nursing center services. *Journal of Community Health Nursing, 4*(1), 29–42.

Baird, S.C., & Benner, R. (1985). Keeping a university well with a health promotion clinic. *Nursing and Health Care, 6,* 107–109.

Barger, S.E. (1985a). Evaluating a nurse-managed center. *Nurse Educator, 10*(4), 36–39.

Barger, S.E. (1985b). Nursing centers: Here today, gone tomorrow? In J.C. McCloskey & H.K. Grace (Eds.), *Current issues in nursing* (2nd ed.) (pp. 752–760). Boston: Blackwell Scientific.

Barger, S.E. (1986a). Academic nurse-managed centers: Issues of implementation. *Family and Community Health, 9*(1), 12–22.

Barger, S.E. (1986b). Nursing center: From concept to reality. *Journal of Community Health Nursing, 3,* 175–182.

Barger, S.E. (1986c). Personnel issues of academic nurse managed centers: The pitfalls and potential. *Nurse Educator, 11*(3), 29–33.

Barger, S.E. (1986d). Academic nursing centers: A demographic profile. *Journal of Professional Nursing, 2,* 246–251.

Barger, S.E. (1987). The potential for resources and research use in academic nurse-managed center. *Nurse Educator, 12,* 19–22.

Benson, E.R., & McDevitt, J.Q. (1978). Know your community resources. *Journal of Gerontological Nursing, 4,* 20–25.

Bloch, D.A. (1985). A conceptualization of nursing research and nursing science. In J.C. McCloskey & H.K. Grace (Eds.), *Current issues in nursing* (2nd ed.) (pp. 130–143). Boston: Blackwell Scientific.

Boettcher, J.M.H. (1986). *A national overview of nurse-managed centers.* Paper presented at the Third Biennial conference on Nurse Managed Centers, Scottsdale, AZ.

Branstetter, E., & Holman, E. (1982). *Billing and record keeping in a nurse-managed center.* Paper presented at the First Biennial Conference on Nurse Managed Centers, Milwaukee, WI.

Brooks, C. (1986). Discontinue care? Nurses say no. In J. Dey, T.R. Misener, & D. Talbot (Eds.), *Community-based nursing services,* American Nurses Association Council of Community Health Nurses, (pp. 3–5). (Available from the American Nurses' Association, 2420 Pershing Rd., Kansas City, MO 64108.)

Brooks, J., & Holle, M.L. (1982). *The Purdue University Nursing Center.* Paper presented at the First Biennial Conference on Nurse Managed Centers, Milwaukee, WI.

Burgess, W. (1988). *The resurgence of nursing centers: 1967–1987.* (Unpublished manuscript available from University of Wisconsin-Milwaukee, School of Nursing, P.O. Box 413, Milwaukee, WI 53201.)

Caspers, B. (1984). *The American Nurses' Association survey of nurse entrepreneurs.* Paper presented at the Second Biennial Conference on Nurse Managed Centers, Milwaukee, WI.

Chickadonz, G.H., Burke, M.M., Fitzgerald, S., Osterweis, M. (1982). Development of a primary care setting for nursing education. *Nursing and Health Care, 3,* 83–87, 92.

Clark, M.J. (1984). Nursing leadership in a shoestring clinic. *Topics in Clinical Nursing, 6*(1), 52–62.

Corcega, T.F. (1982). The partnership approach to health development: Bagong Silangan Nursing Clinic Project. Part I, A case presentation. *ANPHI Papers, 17*, 2–6.

Crane, M.L. (1988). *Erie Family Health Center: A case study.* Paper presented at the Fourth Biennial Conference on Nursing Centers, Milwaukee, WI.

Culang, T.G., Josephson, S.L., Marcus, M.T., & Vezina, M.L. (1980). Implementation of a campus nursing and health center in the baccalaureate curriculum. Part II: Center project health fairs. *Journal of Nursing Education, 19*(5), 11–14.

Culbert-Hinthorn, P., Fiscella, K.D., & Shortridge, L.M. (1985). A nurse-managed clinical practice unit: Part I—The positives. *Nursing and Health Care, 6*, 97–100.

Culbert-Hinthorn, P., Fiscella, K.D., & Shortridge, L.M. (1986). A nurse-managed clinical practice unit: Part II—The problems. *Nursing and Health Care, 7*, 491–494.

Dayani, E.C. (1983). Nursing center bill lets us show what we can do. *The American Nurse, 15*(4), 14.

Dayani, E.C., & Holtmeier, P.A. (1984). Formula for success: A company of entrepreneurs. *Nursing Economics, 2*, 376–381.

Dickerson, P.S., & Nash, B.A. (1985). The business of nursing: Development of a private practice. *Nursing and Health Care, 6,* 327–329.

Duffy, D., & Halloran, M.C. (1987). Effect of an educational program on parents of children with asthma. *Childrens' Health Care, 16*, 76–81.

Duffy, D.M., & Halloran, M.C. (1986). Meeting the challenge of multiple academic roles through a nursing center practice model. *Journal of Nursing Education, 25*, 55–58.

Duvall, A.M., Mural, C.M., & Smith, E.G. (1981). Creative nursing is where you find it: Evolution of a unique nursing clinic. *Nursing Forum, 20*, 167–174.

Ethridge, P. (1987). As I see it . . . Nursing centers make nursing care accessible. *The American Nurse, 19*(1), 5–6.

Fehring, R.J., & Frenn, M. (1986). Nursing diagnosis in a nurse-managed wellness resource center. In M.E. Hurley (Ed.), *Classification of nursing diagnoses: Proceedings of the Sixth Conference* (pp. 401–407). St. Louis: Mosby.

Fehring, R.J., Schulte, J., & Riesch, S.K. (1986). Toward a definition of nurse-managed centers. *Journal of Community Health Nursing, 3*(2), 59–67.

Glass, L.K. (1988). *The historic origins of nursing centers.* Paper presented at the Fourth Biennial Conference on Nursing Centers, Milwaukee, WI.

Gloss, E.F., & Fielo, S.B. (1987). The nursing center: An alternative for health care delivery. *Family and Community Health, 10,* 49–58.

Greshem-Kenton, L., & Wisby, M. (1987). Development and implementation of nurse-managed health program: A problem-oriented approach. *Journal of Ambulatory Care Management, 10*(3), 20–29.

Grimes, D., & Stamps, C. (1980). Meeting the health care needs of older adults through a community nursing center. *Nursing Administration Quarterly, 4,* 31–40.

Grimes, R.E. (1983). Developing neighborhood nurse offices. *Nursing and Health Care, 4,* 138–139.

Hall, L.E. (1963). A center for nursing. *Nursing Outlook, 11,* 805–806.

Hauf, B.J. (1977). An evaluative study of a nursing center for community health nursing student experiences. *Journal of Nursing Education, 16*(8), 7–11.

Hawkins, J.W., Igou, J.F., Johnson, E.E., & Utley, Q.E. (1984). A nursing center for ambulatory, well, older adults. *Nursing and Health Care, 5,* 209–212.

Henry, O.M. (1978, October). *Demonstration centers for nursing practice, education, and research.* Paper presented at the annual meeting of the American Public Health Association, Los Angeles, CA.

Herman, C.M., & Krall, K. (1984). University sponsored home care agency as a clinical site. *Image, 21*(3), 71–75.

Higgs, Z.R. (1985). Carry the water to the desert. *Journal of Professional Nursing, 1,* 217–220.

Hill, J. (1986). Patient evaluation of a rheumatology nursing clinic. *Nursing Times, 82*(27), 42–43.

Jameison, M., & Martinson, I. (1988). *The Block Nurse Program: Neighbors helping neighbors.* Paper presented at the Fourth Biennial Conference on Nursing Centers, Milwaukee, WI.

Johnson, J.C. (1987). Andrea Karlin: Trailblazer in health care. *Northwest Examiner,* p. 20.

Jones, A. (1976). Overview of a nursing center for family health services in Freeport. *Nurse Practitioner, 1*(6), 26–31.

Jones, A., Pagel, I., Wittman, M.E. (1973). Nursing center for family health services. *Journal of New York State Nurses' Association, 4*(1), 33–36.

Kalisch, P.A., & Kalisch, B.J. (1986). *The advance of American nursing* (2nd ed.). Boston: Little, Brown.

Keenan, T. (1984). *Philanthropic support for nurse managed centers.* Paper presented at the Second Biennial Conference on Nurse Managed Centers, Milwaukee, WI.

Kinlein, M.L. (1972). Independent nurse practitioner. *Nursing Outlook, 20,* 22–24.

Kogan, H.N., Beaton, R., Betrus, P., Burr, R., Larson, M.L., Mitchell, P., Wolf-Wilets, V. (1983). Nursing in transition: New structures, new practices, and new consumer responses. *Washington State Journal of Nursing, 54*(2), 37–41.

Kos, B.A., & Rothberg, J.S. (1981). Evaluation of a freestanding nurse clinic. In L.H. Aiken (Ed.), *Health policy and nursing practice* (pp. 19–42). New York: McGraw Hill.

Lamper-Linden, C., Goetz-Kulas, J., & Lake, R. (1983). Developing ambulatory care clinics: Nurse practitioners as primary providers. *The Journal of Nursing Administration, 13,* 11–18.

Lang, N.M. (1983). Nurse-managed centers: Will they thrive? *American Journal of Nursing, 83,* 1290–1293.

Lenehan, G.P., McInnis, B.N., O'Donnell, D., & Hennessey, M. (1985). A nurses' clinic for the homeless. *American Journal of Nursing, 85,* 1237–1240.

Leslie, S., & Houle, M. (1983). Portrait of a nursing center. *Nursing Homes, 32,* 21-27.

Lewis, E.E., & Resnick, B.A. (1967). Nurse clinics and progressive ambulatory patient care. *New England Journal of Medicine, 277*(23), 1236–1241.

Lundeen, S.P. (1985). Editorial: Nurse managed centers offer more to patients, nurses. *The American Nurse, 17,* 4 & 22.

Lyon, B. (in press). An impractical dream or possible reality: A faculty intramural private practice model. In N. Chaska (Ed.), *The nursing profession: Turning points.* St. Louis: Mosby.

Lundeen, S.P. (1986). An interdisciplinary nurse-managed center: The Erie Family Health Center. In M.D. Mezey & D.O. McGivern (Eds.), *Nurses, Nurse Practitioners* (pp. 278–288). Boston: Little, Brown.

MacLeod, R.P. (1984). *The pediatric diagnostic screening center: A working model of a hospital sponsored nurse managed center.* Paper presented at the Second Biennial Conference on Nurse Managed Centers, Milwaukee, WI.

Matthews, J. (1984). College of Nursing outreach: Clinic serves variety of health needs. *Insight, 4*(16), 7–9.

Mezey, M. (1983). Securing a financial base. *American Journal of Nursing, 83*, 1297–1298.

Mezey, M., & Chiamulera, D.N. (1980). Implementation of a campus nursing and health center in the baccalaureate curriculum. Part I: Overview of the center. *Journal of Nursing Education, 19*(5), 7–10.

Milio, N. (1970). *9226 Kerscheval.* Ann Arbor: University of Michigan Press.

Muhlenkamp, A.F., Brown, N.J., & Sands, D. (1985). Determinants of health promotion activities in nursing clinic clients. *Nursing Research, 34*, 327–332.

Munroe, D., & Natale, P. (1982). After-hours call in a primary care nursing practice. *Nurse Practitioner, 7*(5), 24–27.

Newman, J., Sloss, G.S., & Anderson, S. (1984). Evaluation of a health program. *Geriatric Nursing, 5*(6), 234–238.

Nichols, C. (1985a). Faculty practice: Something for everyone. *Nursing Outlook, 33*, 85–90.

Nichols, C.W. (1985b). Postdate pregnancy: Part II clinical implications. *Journal of Nurse-Midwifery, 30*, 259–268.

Nichols, C.W. (1985c). The Yale Nurse Midwifery practice: Addressing the outcomes. *Journal of Nurse-Midwifery, 30*, 159–165.

Norton, S.F., & Nichols, C.W. (1985). Champions of choice. *American Journal of Nursing, 85*, 381–383.

Ossler, C.C., Goodwin, M.E., Mariani, M., & Gilliss, C.L. (1982). Establishment of a nursing clinic for faculty and student clinical practice. *Nursing Outlook, 30*, 402–405.

Pinkava, B.P. (1986). Center benefits students, faculty, and clients. In J. Dey, T.R. Misener, & D. Talbot (Eds.), *Community-based nursing services.* American Nurses' Association Council on Community Health Nurses (72–75). (Available from the American Nurses' Association, 2420 Pershing Rd., Kansas City, MO 64108.)

Resolutions. (1925). *The Kentucky committee for mothers and babies quarterly bulletin, 1*, 15–17.

Riesch, S.K. (1988). Changes in the exercise of self-care agency: childbearing dyad. *Western Journal of Nursing Research, 10*, 257–266.

Riesch, S.K. (1985). A primary care initiative: Nurse-managed centers. In M.D. Mezey & D.O. McGivern (Eds.), *Nurses, Nurse Practitioners* (pp. 242–248). Boston: Little, Brown.

Riesch, S.K., Fehring, R., & Schulte, J. (1987). Expanding the concept of continuing education conferences: The conference participants as a Delphi method sample. *Journal of Continuing Education, 18*(2), 54–58.

Riesch, S.K., & Fehring, R.J. (1986). *The state of the art of research in nursing centers*. Paper presented at the Third Biennial Conference on Nurse Managed Centers, Scottsdale, AZ.

Riesch, S.K., Fehring, R.J., Schulte, J.A., & Wright, N.A. (1986). *State of the art of research in nurse-managed centers*. Paper presented at the Third Biennial Conference on Nursing Centers, Scottsdale, AZ.

Riesch, S.K. (1981). *A survey of existing and planned nurse managed centers among National League of Nursing accredited schools.* (Unpublished manuscript available from S.K. Riesch, UW-Milwaukee, P.O. Box 413, Milwaukee, WI 53211.)

Riesch, S.K., Felder, E., & Stauder, C. (1980). Nursing centers can promote health for individuals, families, and communities. *Nursing Administration Quarterly, 4*(3), 1–8.

Rosenfeld, J. (1984). Nurses called to the rescue. *UCLA Nurse, 2*(1), 10–12.

Ryan, S.A., & Barger-Lux, M.J. (1985). Faculty expertise in a practice—A school succeeding. *Nursing and Health Care, 6*, 75–78.

Sanger, M. (1971). *Margaret Sanger, an autobiography*. New York: Dover. (Reprint of 1938 ed. by W.W. Norton.)

Sheffler, M.V., & Grasse, W.L. (1980). Leader Nursing Center: The goal is rehabilitation and home. *Contemporary Administration, 3*, 10–13.

Smith, E.M. (1986). A nurse-managed family health center at the University of Florida. *Journal of Nursing Education, 25*, 79-81.

Thibodeau, J.A., & Hawkins, J. (1987). Evolution of a nursing center. *Journal of Ambulatory Care Management, 10*(3), 30–39.

Thibodeau, J.A., & Herbert, P.F. (1978). A clinic for senior citizens. *Nurse Practitioner, 3*, 11.

Tsiantar, D. (1986, Sept. 26). Ford Foundation rewards public innovation. *The Washington Post*, A28 & 29.

U.S. Senate (1983, First Session). Community Nursing Centers Act of 1983. S.B. 410, 98th Congress.

Nursing in an Urban Environment

9

TAKING NURSING EDUCATION TO THE STREETS

Dorothy L. Powell, EdD, RN
Dean, College of Nursing
Howard University
Washington, D.C.
Bernardine M. Lacey, MA, RN
Instructor and Project Director
Howard University
Washington, D.C.

Disheveled, unshaven, dirty, smelly, red-eyed drunken men loiter on the sidewalks or park benches and in abandoned buildings. They wear too many clothes and they haul around green plastic bags full of their total poverty-stricken existence. They panhandle for money to support their illicit habits and rampage through garbage cans for discarded food. In the eyes of many, this describes the homeless.

However, that portrait represents only a portion of the growing number of people who are homeless. They are also the elderly, the mentally ill, and the victims of broken homes, abuse and trauma, as well as those who have fallen through the cracks of domestic social programs. The homeless are also pharmacists, lawyers, college professors, veterans, carpenters, electricians, and ministers. They are people who work every day in offices, schools, hospitals, and factories. They consist of families, single women, and children. They are black, white, Hispanic, and all other ethnic groups. These are the homeless and they are drawn from a cross section of America.

Homeless people are prone to a broad array of health problems, complicated by their exposure to environmental extremes, malnutrition, and trauma. Yet they are among those most neglected by the established health care system because of inadequate resources and/or health insurance.

Problems associated with joblessness, unavailable affordable housing, addictive behaviors, broken families, and other overriding social factors form the basis for the health needs of the homeless men, women, and children. The problems of homeless people have grown, but the response of the health care delivery system has lagged behind significantly. There are an estimated 2 to 3 million homeless persons in the United States (HUD, 1984; Hombs & Snyder, 1982) for whom health care services ought to be available. At the very least, providers of health care need to be sensitive to the special needs of homeless people.

The College of Nursing at Howard University in Washington, DC has been particularly sensitive to the homeless problem. In Washington, as in most major cities, evidence of homelessness is an inescapable reality. Rather than be appalled by the situation and retreat to the splendor of the ivy-towered campus, the College of Nursing chose to respond to the crisis in a significant manner. This chapter describes how the undergraduate and graduate nursing programs in this historically black university with its mission of "social uplift" have integrated homelessness into their educational, service, and research activities. We explain how the college became involved, which factors facilitated and impeded our involvement, what we did, and what our future plans are.

HISTORICAL PERSPECTIVE

The college's response to homelessness came about because one faculty member became associated in 1986 with the Community for Creative Non-Violence (CCNV), one of the largest advocacy groups for the homeless. During the mid-1980s, CCNV gained possession of a large vacated federal building for use as a shelter for the city's homeless. A federal appropriation, coupled with some foundation support, provided the needed resources with which to renovate the building as a 1400-bed residential shelter with a health unit in the basement. Our first faculty advocate for the homeless was instrumental in the design of the health unit. It consists of an ambulatory clinic, a 24-bed postdetox unit, and a 32-bed infirmary.

This involvement strengthened the ties between the College of Nursing and CCNV. Equally important, it revealed the vast potential for learning experiences for both the undergraduate and graduate programs. The prospects for health screening, health teaching, and health promotion were numerous. Basic nursing and health assessment skills could be practiced repeatedly, given the volume of potential clients. Opportunities for developing management/leadership and nursing administration skills were possible. The shelter could provide fertile ground for research. The potential for developing problem solving skills was extensive because specific policies and procedures to manage the health care needs of the homeless were lacking. Innovation and critical thinking tools would unquestionably be acquired as the complex problems of the homeless were addressed. Despite the lack of a stable organizational structure, written policies, and protocol, as well as up-to-date equipment and supplies, the shelter environment offered many valuable and challenging learning experiences for students that could be put into perspective by the creative and watchful faculty. The potential positive outcomes envisioned were well worth the risk of the uncertainties and the unknown.

However, winning full faculty support for the integration of homelessness into the fiber of the college's curriculum, community service activities, and research agendas was not without challenges. Preconceptions and uncertainties had to be addressed. Despite the high visibility given to the homeless problem in the media and consciousness raising by nursing organizations such as the National League for Nursing ("Resolution #13," 1987), the internalization of that awareness into a meaningful curricular response by our own nursing education program meant that certain real and perceived impeding factors had to be overcome.

Impeding factors were largely related to curricular issues coupled with concern for the safety of students and faculty. Faculty discussion often reflected such concerns as (1) contentment with the curriculum as existed, (2) a full curriculum leaving no room for additional content and experiences with the homeless, (3) some reluctance to move from a traditional curriculum to one that embraced nontraditional learning experiences, and (4) the lack of history and established guidelines for health care to homeless people. This latter concern was a particularly important one since the infirmary was without a stable staff, and had few written protocols, minimal medical support, few if any nursing role models, a loose organizational structure, and inadequate supplies and equipment. Most of the essentials one looks for when establishing clinical relationships with an agency were missing in the shelter environment. However, the most important resources present were opportunity and people in need of compassion and care. Scores of learning opportunities were evident with each homeless person's situation and within the shelter environment itself.

Another matter that had to be addressed was the question of potential liability of students and faculty. Working with the general counsel for the university, it was determined that the shelter constituted an off-campus clinical site just like all other off-campus sites used by the nursing program. Thus, the same coverage that protected students and faculty engaged in university sanctioned curricula based learning experiences protected them at the shelter as well. It was, however, further deemed that students and faculty engaged in non-class related community service activities were not covered.

This latter understanding did little to resolve the perceived potential danger feared by faculty for their own safety and that of their belongings in an environment where homeless people were thought of as vagrants, drug addicts, and alcoholics. Stereotypic perceptions had to be dispelled and a sense of reasonable precaution had to be instilled. Opportunities for positive exposure to the homeless were determined to be a means of addressing these concerns.

Such opportunities materialized and accounted for one of the major factors that facilitated the integration of homelessness into the graduate and undergraduate programs.

The first opportunity presented itself in 1987 when the city of Washington's Department of Immunization supplied the influenza vaccine to College of Nursing personnel, who administered it to homeless persons prior to the onset of cold weather. The College of Nursing's response came with the planning and implementation of a series of immunization activities targeted primarily at the 1,400 homeless people residing at the federal city shelter. Two evening time periods were arranged for inoculations that would coincide with those times the men congregated at the shelter and/or returned from work. A third time period was planned for the noon hour at a women's shelter. Faculty, graduate students, and clerical staff were recruited to interview, inform, counsel, and inoculate the homeless individuals. In these three short periods, over 700 immunizations were given.

This initial experience accomplished some obvious positive results for the homeless. More importantly, for us, the exposure provided the constituents of the college with a cursory appraisal of who the homeless really are, the variety of health needs that confront them, and the possibilities that exist to provide nursing assistance. Also, all involved in this initial experience came away with a sense of gratification because of the smiles, the receptiveness, and the appreciation shown them by the homeless men and women. The experience also dispelled some of the fears about homeless people and replaced them with understanding and respect for their situation.

Students' satisfaction with opportunities to learn from the homeless and to provide care to them was among the most important factors that facilitated the college's involvement. The initial group of students assigned work with the homeless did so willingly but with the same concerns as many of the faculty. Students, however, were adaptable and quickly became eager learners. Their creativity and problem solving skills were called forth as in no other setting. The students' enthusiasm was contagious and helped faculty to value experiences with the homeless with increasing degrees of satisfaction and approval.

The college's involvement with the homeless gained a lot of attention, initially on campus and later throughout the community as both print and electronic media focused on our work. Increasing public recognition and approval from socially conscious people and colleagues throughout the country reinforced the "rightness" of the college's attempts to redress the problem of homelessness. This in turn generated increasing amounts of internal support and encouraged both curriculum modifications and the teaching/learning process for undergraduate and graduate students.

CURRICULUM BASED HOMELESS EXPERIENCES

Despite the enthusiasm, support, and opportunities which exist, curriculum revision and the related teaching/learning processes are the responsibilities of the faculty. To incorporate a highly visible issue like homelessness into fairly traditional undergraduate and graduate curricula was viewed by faculty with mixed emotions. It was thought of as either an educationally appropriate response to a serious social problem with profound health implications or a risky endeavor plagued with too many uncertainties to be feasible or justifiable at this time. The uncertainties largely resulted from a lack of knowledge about how nursing education could benefit from such an uncharted approach to learning and from the previously discussed personal fears.

Once a few positive encounters were experienced by a significant portion of the faculty and the potentials for meaningful learning were established, curriculum revision gained momentum.

The charge to faculty was to determine which current clinical objectives could be met through rotations at the shelter in the convalescent unit. It was recognized that early experiences might be problematic and certainly challenging. It was further realized that early experiences at the shelter would be of an experimental nature, the results of which would provide valuable feedback to guide the structuring of subsequent experiences.

The junior level course, Health Assessment, was one of the earliest courses to plan a clinical experience in the shelter's 32-bed convalescent unit. Two course objectives were deemed appropriate to guide the clinical experience: (1) to demonstrate beginning skills in performing a physical examination utilizing the techniques of observation, palpation, percussion, and auscultation, and (2) to assess the health status of clients throughout their life spans, considering sociocultural influences and other parameters that promote health or impinge on wellness. Students spent two laboratory days at the shelter on a rotation basis. In implementing their objectives, they were expected to (1) perform physical examinations and report and record findings; (2) assess and analyze health status, discriminating between normal and abnormal findings and interpreting findings in light of the current homeless situations; and (3) identify problems inherent in street living.

An initial orientation to the shelter and the nature of homelessness aided the students' adjustment and sense of well-being. The students' eagerness also contributed to the positive aspect of the experience. However, some difficulties surfaced that challenged faculty, who for the most part had had "hospital" orientations. Facilities for privacy were nonexistent in large ward-like rooms. Equipment and supplies for conducting physicals were not readily available in the facility and had to be loaned by the college. A means for recording and utilizing findings was not in evidence at the shelter. In spite of these limitations, use of the shelter for Health Assessment was appropriate, meaningful, and superior to an on-campus lab in which students assessed each other.

Homeless clients reflected a broad range of normal findings and provided ample opportunities for students to differentiate between normal and abnormal findings. Amidst a wide variety of clients representing rich cultural diversity, the shelter was also an unhurried, casual environment, supportive to young learners. This environment provided a dramatic example through which to explain and analyze the adaptation-based, theoretical framework upon which the curriculum is structured. It also fostered the essential basis for contextual health assessments upon which to formulate appropriate nursing diagnoses for homeless individuals.

Community-Mental Health Nursing, a senior level course, was another of the early undergraduate courses that incorporated the shelter into its clinical experiences. Initial exposure was limited to females only, but later classes gradually included homeless men in the convalescent unit, the postdetoxification unit, and the general residential areas of the mammoth shelter. Out-reach experiences into the residential areas of the shelter gave the students an opportunity to do case finding and health teaching. The faculty considered the shelter one of several clinical sites for the course. One group of students was assigned to the shelter while others went elsewhere. The same objectives governed all clinical sites; thus, the opportunity for comparison and contrast among sites was a valuable learning strategy.

The course objectives and related clinical expectations follow: Students were expected to (1) synthesize theoretical concepts that relate to the health of the community; (2) implement the nursing process with individuals, families, groups, and communities adapting to various levels of stress; and (3) function as a change agent while providing nursing care in the community. In implementing these objectives, students assessed the community of the homeless, identifying those factors that facilitate and impede healthy adaptation. Further, students were expected to conduct case findings by making rounds in the shelter and to provide comprehensive nursing care, health promotion, and health teaching activities for individuals and groups. Moreover, students had the opportunity to act as resource persons and catalysts, to assist in identifying priorities for health promotion and health maintenance activities for the homeless community, and to advocate for the homeless. Students and faculty believed the experience facilitated innovation, creativity, and problem solving.

The success of the first courses inspired additional nursing courses during the second year to identify ways that their clinical learning needs could be obtained at least in part at the shelter. Medical-Surgical Nursing, a junior level course, adopted the shelter as an additional site for a course that had depended exclusively on acute care facilities. The inclusion strengthened the health promotion and health teaching aspects of the course. The same objectives, with minor modifications, that guide the course and its related clinical practice were deemed appropriate for the shelter setting. These included (1) application of the nursing process to clients with altered health states, including impaired peripheral circulation, selected hormonal imbalances, and impaired CO_2-O_2 exchange; (2) use of culturally relevant, innovative approaches in seeking solutions to altered health states among diverse groups of people; (3) participation as a member of a multidisciplinary health team; and (4) engaging in activities that foster the health promotion and maintenance capabilities of clients.

The types of clients that could satisfy the objectives were in large number at the shelter. The typical homeless person admitted to the convalescent unit might have gangrene, leg ulcers, diabetes, respiratory impairment as well as other problems because of exposure, trauma, and malnutrition. The group was culturally diverse and came from every strata of society, race, and educational background. During these experiences, students had opportunities to confer with other health professionals, such as physicians or physician assistants. Students were also expected to design and conduct health promotion classes for the homeless and staff development activities for the volunteer staff at the shelter.

Another major objective of the course was to collaborate with members of the health team while providing a variety of services to people. In implementing this objective, senior students collaborated with graduate students to design, implement, and evaluate a health fair for the homeless that provided health teaching, health screening, and other health promotion activities. Students gained valuable knowledge concerning the vast array of community agencies and services needed to implement the health fair. Coordinating skills were developed through the orchestration of all aspects of the fair. Leadership and advocacy role development were additional benefits of the experience.

The fourth undergraduate course to elect to incorporate homelessness into its curriculum was Essential Components of Nursing. This sophomore level fundamentals of nursing course had a tradition of focusing on the attainment of skills in a hospital setting. The faculty's decision to alter the experiences to include the shelter as a major clinical site underscored a broadening perspective of the faculty; that is, a movement beyond skills to a focus on problem solving and the enhanced application of theory-based practice. Two of the course objectives were considered suitable for fulfillment at the shelter: (1) describe adaptive behaviors which represent how people organize and integrate their environment to prevent disturbances of function and (2) apply the nursing process to selected client situations.

In addressing the first objective, the conceptual framework of the college was critically analyzed in light of the impact of the external environment and adaptive behaviors in the cognitive, personal, and physical domains. Through interviews, observations, and assessments, students were able to operationalize the conceptual framework. Students also compared and contrasted their findings with classmates who had similar experiences in another, more traditional long-term care facility. In the achievement of this objective, students also practiced communicative and interpersonal skills.

The second objective allowed students to gain experience with the various phases of the nursing process. Ample opportunities were available to assess vital signs, skin, mental status, developmental level, etc. Interpretation of findings was in light of accepted norms but with an acute awareness of life style and environmental circumstances. Planning and implementation were possible for a variety of nursing diagnoses, followed by the application of interventional strategies such as dressing changes, range of motion, hot and cold applications, exercise, foot care, the maintenance of a clean and therapeutic environment, and health teaching. Lastly, students were guided in evaluating the effectiveness of their interventions. Because many clients were long term in the convalescent unit, students could frequently see changes from week to week.

Graduate students have also been integrally involved with homelessness in several of their graduate majors and role development areas. The college recently phased out a major in Nursing Administration and replaced it with an administration role development area in association with the three majors: Adult Health, Gerontology, or Primary Family Health. The original administrative major focused much of its clinical application on addressing administrative issues within the context of a nontraditional health care delivery system. Hence, the emerging system of health care at the shelter proved to be a challenging and valuable experience. One advantage of the shelter was that students were involved in the initial creation of standards, policies, and protocols— and then had the opportunity to test them. Problem solving by applying resolution strategies, including a focus on establishing controls, was one of the possible learning activities for graduate students.

The focus on homelessness was continued with administration as a role development area. Similar experiences were incorporated into the administrative role development track as had been evident with the administration major. The following objectives framed the homeless experience and were added to those individually set by students: (1) analyze selected organizational environments in relation to administrative and management theory, identifying areas needing administrative intervention, and (2) apply administrative theory and management principles in the identification of a broad organizational or systematic problem and design, organize, implement, control, and evaluate a nursing response to the identified need.

Within the context of the shelter's philosophy, which values self-care, volunteerism, and sharing, students conducted in-depth analyses of the current and projected health services and identified areas needing managerial intervention. Students proposed, planned, implemented, and evaluated their managerial interventions. Many of their suggestions were incorporated into the evolving organizational structure of the shelter.

FUTURE PLANS

The future of the College of Nursing's involvement with the homeless is promising. A recent 3-year, million dollar grant from the W. K. Kellogg Foundation will enable the college to develop and test a nurse-managed model for health care delivery that focuses on health promotion, health maintenance, and convalescent care. The model will demonstrate how a shelter staff of registered nurses and nurse practitioners, nursing students, faculty, volunteer staff, and other health professionals can work together to extend health care to the homeless while at the same time providing a meaningful and sensitizing experience for students.

In addition, the project will identify and train selected homeless individuals to serve in assistant roles in the infirmary. It is envisioned that curriculum development, teaching, and evaluation for these trainees will constitute valuable learning experiences for graduate students in the educator role development track. Similarly, graduate students in the administration track should benefit from the selection, orientation, supervision, inservice training, evaluation, and subsequent assistance in placement of health assistants who seek gainful employment.

We plan to develop audiovisual media that will address the needs both of the homeless and of health professionals. Health promotion videos that are the result of the collaborative wisdom of homeless persons, project personnel, and students will be produced to assist homeless persons to improve and/or maintain health in the face of their deprived existence. In addition, films that chronicle the evolution of homelessness as part of nursing students' educational experiences should be a resource for other schools of nursing and interested groups.

The challenges of working with the homeless and impacting on the status of their health are many. The benefits to students, faculty, and the curriculum are evident. Above all, the experiences have allowed the college to respond to the needs of society as it strives to make nursing education relevant, challenging, and dynamic.

REFERENCES

Hombs, M.E., & Snyder, M. (1982). *Homelessness in America: A forced march to nowhere*. Washington, DC: Community for Creative Non-Violence.

National League for Nursing Resolution #13: Adopted by the NLN membership at the 18th biennial Convention. (1987). *Nursing and Health Care, 8,* September.

U.S. Department of Housing and Urban Development (HUD) (1984). *A report to the Secretary on the homeless and emergency shelters*. Washington, DC: Office of Policy Development and Research.

10

COMMUNITY HEALTH ADVOCACY: PRIMARY HEALTH CARE NURSE-ADVOCATE TEAMS IN URBAN COMMUNITIES

Beverly J. McElmurry, EdD, FAAN
Professor
Susan M. Swider, PhD, RN
Project Co-director
Cathy Bless, RN, MPH
Community Nurse
Dorothy Murphy, BSN, RN
Community Nurse
Andy Montgomery, PhD
Sociologist/Database Development

Kathleen Norr, PhD
Sociologist/Evaluator
Yvonne Irvin, PhD
Psychologist
Margaret Gantes, MS, RN
Doctoral Student/Evaluation
Marlene Fisher, MS, RN
Doctoral Student/Database
College of Nursing
University of Illinois at Chicago
Chicago, Illinois

OVERVIEW: WOMEN'S HEALTH EXCHANGE

The notion of collaborating with patients/clients in the process of planning and designing health care services is familiar to community health practitioners and is even becoming less of a novelty for hospital-based practice in this era of "marketing" our so-called health care product. But for those of us who are based in an academic setting, where research development is the number one priority, getting out into the community to test the wind and, then, to design appropriate health care programs, is easier said than done.

The Women's Health Exchange of the College of Nursing, University of Illinois at Chicago, includes students and faculty with a strong interest in and commitment to women's health. With representation from each of the five departments within the College of Nursing (Medical-Surgical, Community Health, Maternal-Child, Psychiatry, and Administrative Studies in Nursing), our collaboration began in 1977 when a research interest group was formed within the college as a means of fostering research in women's health. That initial effort was stimulated by a federal grant, the Doctoral Expansion Grant, entitled *Building Nursing Knowledge* (DON, HEW, Grant #1 D23-NU0093).

Since its inception in 1977, the Women's Health Group has sustained a high degree of collegiality and productivity as the following list of accomplishments illustrates:

1979: Research Development Workshop, *Women's Health: An Exchange of Ideas*. Representatives of over 50 community women's groups participated in this grass-roots endeavor to identify and discuss research possibilities in women's health. The proceedings were printed and made available to participants (Mackey, 1980).

1979: Outreach to practitioners in nursing. This initiative was in the form of a series of consultation sessions with small groups of clinical specialists whose interests included public health, midwifery, psychiatric nursing, breast cancer, parenting, and substance abuse.

1981: Establishment of a resource center known as the Women's Health Exchange. This resource center contains books, files of health education materials, periodicals, annotated bibliographies, and some audiovisual materials.

1982: Development of the Women's Health Advocacy Training Program. With funding from the University of Illinois Urban Health Program and the City of Chicago, faculty provided 145 hours of training for 26 minority women between the ages of 17 and 21. Training consisted of classroom sessions, field placements, group counseling, field trips, and independent assignments in subject matter such as basic health practices, child abuse, substance abuse, aging, mental health, assertiveness training, health skills for parents, self-defense, self-help, and health promotion.

1984: Beginning of 5 years of support to develop the Graduate Nursing Concentration in Women's Health (#1 D23-NU00455). This project was designed to develop a curriculum that emphasizes research training in women's health. Courses and seminars have been presented to address theory development, methods in women's health research, and issues and controversies in the field of women's health. Since its inception, the Graduate Nursing Concentration in Women's Health has attracted an increasing number of students with a serious interest in women's health.

1987: Received funding from the Chicago Community Trust to conduct health advocacy training and community assessment programs. This project further developed the 1982 project and is the project described in this presentation.

1989: Received funding from the Kellogg Foundation to demonstrate collaborative decision making in Primary Health Care with community residents and health professionals.

Concurrent with the above funded projects, many of our students have had individual, federal, and foundation support grants for their doctoral study. Overall,

Women's Health refers to the nursing care of women within the context in which they live their lives. The roles and socio-economic conditions of women are interdependent and influence their health or illness status. A study concentration in women's health provides an opportunity for students to learn about women's life experiences from multiple perspectives: historical, political, cultural, developmental, and socio-economic. An awareness of the variability of women's experiences provides the background a student uses to understand a client's view of her situation. To this end, the provision of health care and the formulation of research questions that benefit women are those which arise from women's lived experiences. Women's health is concerned with women both as consumers and providers of health care—in multiple settings, and while assuming changing roles. As women's life experiences change, so will education, nursing care, and research in women's health. (Webster & Lipetz, 1986 - adapted.)[1] The authors gratefully acknowledge the influence of work done by McBride & McBride (1981).

HEALTH IN THE INNER CITY

Low-income, urban communities in the United States illustrate a variety of disparate health problems. These problems range from the chronic, lifestyle-related conditions found in developed countries to the acute illnesses attributable to conditions of malnutrition, poor sanitation, and inadequate housing more commonly found in developing countries. Low-income community residents need assistance to change the social conditions leading to the acute illnesses as well as the ongoing medical care needed to treat chronic illnesses. Unfortunately, health services in urban areas are focused on the medical treatment of illnesses and low-income people often find it difficult to access these services.

Further, the low levels of formal education in the low income populations often result in inability to adequately use existing services. The detrimental health effects of such factors as stress due to poverty, substance abuse, crime, and poor housing result in a situation where the people least educated (or otherwise equipped to understand health promotion and disease treatment) live in the most hazardous environments with the least health services.

There will be little change in health care of low income groups in the United States as long as nurses and other health care providers continue to treat the specific illnesses of low-income individuals without consideration of the community factors and dynamics which have an effect on their health status. Conversely, community residents are well aware of the dynamics and environment of their neighborhood, yet they lack understanding of the health issues created by that environment.

The thesis of our work is that if the health problems found in low-income, urban communities are to be addressed, the community residents must be empowered to assume appropriate self-care responsibilities and to help shape community responses to their health needs. Concurrently, health providers must learn to view human health and illness within the context of an interaction of social and health conditions. An approach to health services that addresses the importance of this social-health interaction and collaboration between health providers and community residents is primary health care.

PHC FRAMEWORK

There have been few reports in the literature of United States health services based on the concept of *primary health care* (PHC). In this respect the project we describe offers a unique nursing practice demonstration project based on PHC. The definition of PHC we use is the following World Health Organization (WHO) statement:

> Primary health care is essential health care based on practical, scientifically sound and socially acceptable methods and technology made universally accessible to individuals and at a cost that the community and country can afford to maintain at every stage of their development in the spirit of self–reliance and self-determination (WHO, 1978).

We assume that a PHC emphasis in the United States has not been enthusiastically embraced because many health providers and policy makers see it as more appropriate for developing countries. In a health care system that emphasizes advanced technology for the care of illness and disease, it is not surprising that health professionals in the United States have been slow to embrace PHC, a health strategy requiring a major conceptual shift in the definition of comprehensive, quality health services.

The health literature illustrates that major declines in morbidity and mortality in developed countries are related more to social change than to improved medical care (McKinlay & McKinlay, 1977; McKinlay, 1979; McKeown, 1976). For example, McKnight (1978) conducted a study in a Chicago West side neighborhood and found that the seven most common reasons for hospitalization were related to social problems rather than to disease. As Mahler (1981) explained several years ago, the WHO goal of health for all does not mean that all people should have all existing ailments repaired and that no one would be sick or disabled. Rather, Mahler continued, health should be considered in the broader context of its contribution to, and promotion by, social and economic development. We find the PHC perspective appropriate for the United States and the urban health crisis. This perspective will be illustrated throughout our presentation.

PERSPECTIVE ON WOMEN'S HEALTH

In the United States, the goals of the women's health movement are consistent with PHC. Much of the women's health literature focuses on the importance of understanding the lived experience of women (McBride & McBride, 1981). This concept stresses the need to attend to the daily experiences and perceptions of women and then to use these perceptions as a starting point for assessing and planning for the health of women. Such an understanding requires communication between health providers and consumers. While such communication is consistent with the PHC focus on collaboration to plan for community health, the women's health focus has often taken an individualistic focus, whereas PHC is community focused. Our discussions of PHC and women's health is consistent with the following assumptions:

1. The human body, mind, and spirit form an integrated whole.

2. People have capacity for self-care and self-healing.

3. Events and interactions in the family, community, and the world affect and shape the health of people.

4. Health care is the shared responsibility of society, the health care system, and the individual.

5. Health reflects integrity, flexibility, the capacity to develop, and the capacity to creatively transcend difficult situations.

6. Control over one's body is a basic right.

7. Women's life experiences are the starting point for future action.

8. Women's health care practice can take place in a variety of settings, including ambulatory care clinics, communities, hospitals, and universities.

9. By focusing on women, health care for all will be improved; men are not excluded as either providers or recipients. (Chicago School of Thought in Women's Health, 1986)

Further, our discussion of PHC and women's health is consistent with the history of nurses in community-based health care focused on the social health interactions of and in collaboration with community residents. In the 1920s Lillian Wald (1927) structured a nursing practice based on reaching out to poverty-stricken populations and acknowledging the social precursors of illness. Wald worked to help communities provide health-promoting opportunities for children, through improved nutrition, fresh air, and a chance for physical activity. She also worked for changes in social policies relevant to health, such as declaring child labor illegal while legalizing contraceptive methods for women. In the 1970s, Nancy Milio (1970) described collaborative work with low income Detroit neighborhood residents that improved child care and related health activities and documented the process of helping a community plan, develop, and maintain health related programs.

In the project described here—health advocacy in two low-income Chicago communities—the PHC emphasis integrates the ideas of community level change, social-health interaction, a broad definition of health, and a core of essential health services. In essence, it is a test of the PHC approach with the complex health problems found in urban, low income communities of North America.

COMMUNITY HEALTH ADVOCACY PROJECT

The essential aspect of our Community Health Advocacy Project is the development of a team composed of community health advocates and a nurse, who collaborate in defining, developing, and implementing strategies responsive to the concerns and essential health needs of community residents. Elsewhere, we have described the origin of the project (McElmurry, et al., 1987) as a desire to teach basic health promotion behaviors to low-income women. In our initial effort, a curriculum was designed to teach health advocacy. An advocate was defined as a person from the community who shared basic health information with the community and helped community residents make and implement health decisions: a role akin to that of a community health worker. When this curriculum was presented again in 1986 to women hired to conduct case finding of mothers and infants at risk in a nearby public housing project, we learned a little more about health advocacy. One of the frustrations expressed by these community women was that the people in their area had multiple health and social problems that could not be addressed by case finding or advocacy work limited to pregnant women and new mothers. In both of our early projects we had little contact with the women after the training period ended.

Our current project began in 1987 in response to a request for innovative proposals to address the health needs of underserved groups in Chicago. Our intent was to prepare women from two low-income communities in Chicago as health advocates who would work in their communities in collaboration with a public health nurse. For this project our earlier curriculum was revised to include a basic health emphasis, job skills orientation, and periodic meetings with a psychologist to work on skills in communication, conflict resolution, and interpersonal relationships. The training program began with classroom instruction on a variety of health topics, followed by a community health assessment experience in which the nurse-advocate team in each community assessed residents' perceptions of health problems and community health resources. In the subsequent evolution of the advocacy program, this assessment has been used as a basis for planning and implementing nurse-advocate team activities which are acceptable to the community residents and consistent with their PHC concerns.

DESCRIPTION OF COMMUNITIES

The Community Health Advocacy Project has been implemented in two low-income communities in Chicago, one primarily black and the other largely Hispanic.

Grand Boulevard, on Chicago's near South side, is a small community area of 50,000 residents, over 99% of whom are black. This community is home to several public housing projects, most notably Robert Taylor Homes, the largest public housing complex in the world. Grand Boulevard is comprised of young families, 43% of which are headed by single women. It has an unemployment rate of 24% and 56% of its population lived below the poverty line in 1980. The community is characterized by an infant mortality rate of 21.5/1,000 live births; a rate of sexually transmitted diseases of 26.1/100,000 pop., which is 2.6 times that in Chicago as a whole; a homicide rate of .77/1,000 pop., which is almost three times greater than the overall Chicago rate; rampant substance abuse; crime; high incidence rates of communicable diseases; and an absence of health and social services. This is the community that

University of Chicago sociologist Julius Wilson refers to in his book, *The Truly Disadvantaged* (1987).

By contrast, West Town is a large area on Chicago's Northwest side with a population comprised of primarily Hispanic and Eastern European immigrants. West Town has infant mortality rates (15.8/1,000 live births) as well as illness rates and crime and poverty rates (31% of pop. below poverty level) higher than Chicago as a whole but not as high as for Grand Boulevard. However, the community has a large population of illegal immigrants and a language barrier that prevents many residents from seeking health care.

PROJECT ACTIVITIES

Women from each community were selected for training as health advocates with the help of local, social, and health agencies collaborating with our project. The advocates' initial classroom training component consisted of 160 hours of community health education, job/problem solving/advocacy skills development, and field work. Classes were taught by project staff, faculty, and graduate students at the College of Nursing as well as local health and social service workers.

After the training component was completed, the advocates began working in their communities in collaboration with the public health nurses. In the first year, the nurse-advocate teams worked to identify health problems in their community, talk to community residents about health concerns, and assess the health and social services available to meet these needs. As the nurse-advocate team worked out of the community sites and met at the College of Nursing once a week to share experiences, the project staff gathered data on health status indicators for each community in a more traditional community assessment process. Our products here were the assessments of each community, listing both perceived problems and available agencies. To develop the consumer guides to the health and social services in the communities, the project staff and the advocates developed an assessment format and visited each site to determine the nature and type of services provided.

As the assessment phase of the project implementation continued, it became apparent that the advocates were obtaining information not usually obtained by health professionals. The health problems identified in the community were not problems typically addressed by health providers. Community residents were primarily concerned with such social issues and systemic problems as: housing; crime; availability of nutritious, inexpensive food; and lack of good quality medical care. These problems expressed by the residents were concerns about the basic needs of individuals that affected their health. The nurse-advocate teams were responsive to the community residents with whom they lived and worked, and the emerging concerns reflected health and social needs characteristic of a broad definition of health.

To operationalize the community collaboration characteristic of PHC, the advocates and project staff developed an interview guide to survey community residents' health concerns. The guide was based on the eight essential elements of PHC: health education; proper nutrition; safe water and basic sanitation; maternal-child health care, including family planning; immunizations; treatment of common diseases and injuries; prevention and control of endemic diseases; and provision of essential drugs. The advocates used this guide to interview residents and then brought the results back to the larger group for discussion.

By the end of the first year, the advocates had formulated a list of priority health concerns in their community, based upon their work with residents. In addition, the project staff collected statistical health indicators around this priority list, i.e., statistics reflecting community concerns identified by the advocates.

COMMUNITY PRIORITIES

The prioritized list of community health problems the advocates in both communities developed, based on their experiences and their discussions with other residents (Community Health Advocacy Project, 1987), included the following.

Parental Stress. Both communities have large proportions of families headed by single women.

Substance Abuse. Both communities have high rates of substance abuse and related criminal activity.

Teen Pregnancy. Both communities have high proportions of unmarried teen mothers with related income problems, low birth weight infants, and high infant mortality rates.

Lack of Good Quality Medical Services. In both communities, Medicaid clinics are prevalent and known throughout the neighborhoods as places where drug therapy is pushed. One hospital in Grand Boulevard closed during the first project year. Both communities have Chicago Department of Health clinics with family planning services. The city hospital most accessible to people without funds is the County Hospital, and it is some distance from both communities. In West Town the cooperating community based health services agency provides quality medical care for part of the community. Dental services and mental health services are almost nonexistent in both communities.

Nutrition. Community residents have little knowledge of good nutrition. In addition, the Grand Boulevard community has no major food stores. The smaller stores within walking distance charge two to three times more for food than the larger, major chain food stores.

Mental Health. Crowded living conditions, poverty, and unemployment add to stress levels.

Crime. Both community areas are centers of gang and drug activity with crime rates three to four times that of the city in general. In Grand Boulevard, homicide was the fourth leading cause of death in 1983.

Domestic Violence. Residents relate numerous stories of beatings and sexual assault. The advocates in West Town found no services available for such victims. In Grand Boulevard there is one shelter for abused women.

There is much overlap in the listing of community problems. For example, crime is related to substance abuse, and both affect mental health. Some services exist to meet the needs identified here, but community residents are often either unaware of them or have problems getting access to the services which do exist. Many of these problems, and the resultant health effects, require fundamental social change, not merely medical treatment.

CURRENT NURSE-ADVOCATE TEAM ACTIVITIES

In addition to the first year assessment activities, the nurse-advocate team performed some individual advocacy functions for those in need of referral for health and social problems. In the second year, they have increased the provision of such services and developed plans to address the most pressing community health needs identified in the assessment process. By focusing on targeted community health needs, the teams are better able to assess the outcomes of their work.

The nurse-advocate teams perform a variety of health education and networking functions, often at the request of other community groups. These activities include classes in first-aid for children, well-child care, parental support groups, hypertension and breast cancer screening, AIDS education, and nutrition classes. In large part, their current efforts emphasize parenting issues, the primary concern identified in both communities. However, the nurse-advocate teams also respond to requests for health programs from various agencies and thus bring a health focus to groups that would otherwise not have the resources to address health issues.

Most of the advocacy work to date has focused on the individual or institutional level. However, as the nurse-advocate teams become better established in each community, they are better able to identify community level health activities. An example of aggregate level activity is seen in the advocates who have become involved with housing issues and groups acting to improve public housing conditions in the complex that contains one of our offices. The advocates are developing activities that attract the involvement of larger numbers of community residents.

Methods to stimulate community interest include door-to-door canvassing to advertise workshops and elicit resident opinions. Now in the planning stage and designed to compare community participation is a community forum, during which the teams present the community assessments and their ideas for dealing with health priorities to groups of community residents. Through health forums, the teams intend to obtain community confirmation of the identified priorities as well as feedback about the ideas for resolution of the identified priorities. At this time, the advocate teams are conducting mobile health fairs—short health information programs presented at shopping centers, parks, and housing developments.

EVALUATION

Documenting change in a community is a challenging issue. In projects of this sort, documenting community change as a result of our efforts has been a major concern. By the end of the first year we were documenting changes in our staff and advocates and the quality of data collected. To be true to our collaborative PHC ideals, we did not predetermine the problems of mutual concern to the community and the nurse-advocate teams.

In the process of developing evaluation measures, we have studied the Pan American Health Organization (PAHO) (1987) prospective analysis methodology for projecting desired changes in nursing education and services to realize PHC goals. The PAHO perspective uses the organizing categories of context, structure, function, and integrity to examine elements of PHC. We found these categories helpful for evaluation purposes and structured our approach accordingly. In the evaluation format we devised within each category, PHC concepts are defined, program elements specified, and indicators established to represent the qualitative and quantitative evaluation elements desired. Our evaluation plan for this project allows us to examine both the process and the outcome of our activities to facilitate empowerment of community residents in relation to social-health interactions and desired changes.

We document the numbers of community people who become involved in our various activities and the types of activities we conduct: workshops, individual encounters, community meetings, etc. Using the evaluation format we also collect some qualitative data on the process of problem solving by the nurse-advocate teams. We remain realistic about expected measures of change in the community, in part because of the comprehensive, broad-based approach we are taking to community health and in part because the communities we work within are so problem-ridden that a modest effort such as ours is unlikely to make an appreciable dent in the commonly collected statistics.

Our efforts to develop collaborative activities between the university and community members have many interesting challenges. Although the faculty, students, and staff have over 10 years of experience working in both of our target communities, our credibility and commitment to the community continues to be challenged. This is not an entirely unfair accusation—major universities have education and research priorities, which do not reward long-term service activities. Yet, many of the creative ideas of experts who reside in universities require access to real settings for these ideas to be tested. Finding means for the academic community to access the targeted communities for this project is a two-way process that enhances availability of university resources to communities which traditionally have little access to university personnel. Ideally, the university can share ideas, help test them out, and then take a consultative role for further implementation and evaluation. This project is an example of the university/community collaborative process.

This past year we added master's degree students in public health nursing to our project. They were included for a 3-quarter practicum experience (1 credit/quarter), focusing on the assessment, planning, and evaluation of community health programs. In essence, we made the project available as a clinical practice site, but we did not participate in designing the theory sequence which the students take concurrently with the student practicum. We could write an entire paper on what we learned in this aspect of the project. We had very positive experiences for the most part and all participants grew in self-knowledge and knowledge of others. We also learned valuable lessons in clinical teaching, building trust, dealing with racism, accessing physically unsafe environments, and facing professional imperialism. We would like to see students continue to work with the project for practicum as well as research/evaluation experiences. We would also like to see more emphasis on PHC as a perspective that is important in community health nursing education and preparation for practice in low-income urban settings.

LESSONS LEARNED AND CHALLENGES AHEAD

The Community Health Advocacy Project has served to encourage community participation in problem solving as well as increase community involvement in health decisions and community knowledge about health care. Our focus on the health and social interaction involved in satisfying essential health needs and our collaboration with communities to define needs and strategies is consistent with the WHO primary health care approach. It is difficult to achieve true collaboration with community residents. Nurses must resist the tendency to believe they are the experts. Learning to listen to community residents provides the basis for developing a trust relationship between the advocates, the community, and the staff. But it takes time to build trust relationships in general and especially in specific cases where you are identified with a university system that is perceived as not being particularly responsive to minority populations. Thus, we must constantly find ways to demonstrate the worth of the university to the community and help community residents access and use the university resources. Overall, our focus on empowerment means teaching and encouraging people to problem solve for community change related to the provision of primary health care.

SUMMARY

In summary, our health advocacy program uses PHC teams in urban, underserved communities to deal with the interaction of social and health factors in solving problems related to access to appropriate (as perceived by residents) and affordable health care. This approach encourages grass-roots participation in problem identification and solution, a fundamental ingredient of community empowerment. Further, this program facilitates community identification of nurses as resource persons who encourage collaboration to improve the community's health status and as health providers who enhance the authority and autonomy of community participation in the resolution of health issues.

ACKNOWLEDGEMENTS

The authors wish to acknowledge the contributions of Mary Ann Rayford–Marion, RN; and Ellen Barton, MS, RN, to this project. Also, we are grateful for the ongoing support and advice of the Women's Health Group, UIC, CON, especially Alice Dan, PhD; Diane Boyer, PhD, RN, CNM; Diana Biordi, PhD, RN; and Barbara Logan, PhD, RN. The project values the cooperation of Centers for New Horizons and Erie Family Health Center, both in Chicago, IL. We could not continue our efforts without the hard work and energy of our Community Health Advocates: Mary Bell, Carlotta Hill, Cheryl Love, Sharon Martin, Evelia Medina, Diana Robinson, Mildred Rodriguez, Margarita Rosado, and Juanita Tate.

REFERENCES

Chicago School of Thought in Women's Health (D. Webster, L. Leslie, B. McElmurry, A. Dan, D. Biordi, D. Boyer, S. Swider, H. Lipetz, & J. Newcomb) (1986). Concept paper: Nursing practice in women's health. *Nursing Research, 35*, 143.

Community Health Advocacy Project (1987). *Community Health Assessment for Grand Boulevard/West Town.* Unpublished documents. Chicago: University of Illinois, College of Nursing.

Mackey, M. (Ed.). (1980). *Proceedings, women's health research: An exchange of ideas.* Chicago: University of Illinois, College of Nursing.

Mahler, H. (1981). The meaning of "Health for all by the year 2000." *World Health Forum, 2,* 5–22.

McBride, A.B., & McBride, W.L. (1981). Theoretical underpinnings for women's health. *Women & Health, 6,* 37–55.

McElmurry, B.J., Swider, S.M., Grimes, M.J., Dan, A.J., Irvin, Y.S., & Lourenco, S.V. (1987). Health advocacy for young, low-income, inner-city women. *Advances in Nursing Science, 9,* 62–75.

McKeown, T. (1976). *The role of medicine: Dreams, mirage or nemesis.* London: Nuffield Provincial Hospitals Trust.

McKinlay, J.B., & McKinlay, S.M. (1977). The questionable contribution of medical measures to the decline of mortality in the United States in the twentieth century. *Milbank Memorial Fund Quarterly, 53,* 405–428.

McKinlay, J.B. (1979). Epidemiological and political determinants of social policies regarding the public health. *Social Science & Medicine, 13A,* 541–558.

McKnight, J.L. (1978). Politicizing health care. *Social Policy,* Nov.-Dec., 36–39.

Milio, N. (1970). *9226 Kercheval—The storefront that did not burn.* Ann Arbor: University of Michigan Press.

Pan American Health Organization (1987). Prospective analysis methodology for primary health care. Unpublished document. Washington, DC: Author.

Wald, L. (1927). *The house on Henry Street.* New York: Holt.

Webster, D., Leslie, L., McElmurry, B.J., Dan, A., Biordi, D., Boyer, D., Swider, S., Lipetz, M., & Newcomb, J. (1986). Nursing practice in women's health—A concept paper. In Letters to the Editor. *Nursing Research, 35*(3), 143; and *JOGNN, 15*(3), 273.

Webster, D.B., & Lipetz, M. (1986). Changing times: Changing definitions. *Nursing Clinics of North America, 21,* 87–98.

Wilson, W.J. (1987). *The truly disadvantaged: The inner city, the underclass, and public policy.* Chicago: University of Chicago Press.

World Health Organization. (1978). *Primary Health Care.* Geneva, Switzerland: Author.

Nursing Homes

11

THE COMMUNITY COLLEGE–NURSING HOME PARTNERSHIP: IMPROVING CARE THROUGH EDUCATION

Verle Waters, MA, RN
Project Administrator and Assistant Dean of Instruction
Ohlone College
Fremont, California

This W. K. Kellogg (WKK)–funded project can be considered a companion to the Robert Wood Johnson (RWJ) Teaching Nursing Home project. The Community College–Nursing Home Partnership project targets associate degree nursing education; the RWJ project targeted baccalaureate and graduate education. Our nursing home partners are community nursing homes, mostly small, many part of a for-profit chain of nursing homes. RWJ teaching nursing homes are generally large, close to major medical centers. RWJ emphasized research; WKK focuses on bedside skills and patient-care management.

Each year nearly 60% of the new nurses graduate from associate degree programs, beginning careers that will reach well into the next century (National League for Nursing, 1988). Robert Butler points out that students entering the health professions today will spend 75% of their worklife taking care of patients over 65 (Robert Butler, M.D., personal communication, January 27, 1988). This "demographic imperative," the continuing increase in the percentage of the over-65 population, is reshaping health care services. In particular, the over-85 group, the fastest growing segment of our population, are heavy users of nursing care (National Center for Health Statistics, 1987). In 1985, for example, for every 1,000 of our citizenry as a whole, 954 days of hospital care were needed (National Center for Health Statistics, 1987). For every 1,000 citizens 75 years of age or older, 4,389 days of hospital care were needed (National Center for Health Statistics, 1987). Half of the residents in the nation's 19,000 nursing homes are 85 years of age or older.

These facts led us to conclude that the curriculum of the associate degree program must prepare its graduates for nursing the elderly, and for nursing roles in long-term care settings as well as acute care.

That became the major purpose of our project.

Another aspect is to develop the community nursing home as an effective placement for clinical education for nursing students. With nearly 800 associate degree nursing (ADN) programs scattered through the cities and towns of every state, and 19,000 nursing homes similarly distributed, if every nursing program developed an educational partnership with two, three, or four nursing homes in its own community, it could have an impact (National League for Nursing, 1988).

To meet these two purposes, we set forth five specific objectives:

1. Communication and cooperation to create links and active relationships between associate degree nursing programs and providers of health care services to the elderly—especially nursing homes.

2. Inservice training programs for staff development in the nursing home as part of developing a climate for clinical education of basic students.

3. Curriculum change to increase and improve instruction in geriatric/long-term care nursing.

4. Stimulate community college faculty interest and involvement in the field of gerontology and the health care of the aged.

5. Foster in students positive attitudes toward older adults, and encourage graduate interest in geriatric nursing as a career choice.

Six demonstration sites have been meeting those two purposes through an array of activities. The demonstration sites are: Community College of Philadelphia; Shoreline Community College, Seattle; Triton College, in River Grove, a Chicago suburb; Valencia Community College, Orlando, FL; Weber State College, Ogden, UT, a statewide ADN program; and Ohlone College, in the East Bay area of San Francisco.

Project activities at each demonstration site reflect the individuality of each college and its community, but the following core activities are going on in each place:

1. Faculty development. Since its inception, the associate degree nursing curriculum has focused on acute care; it follows that as a group ADN faculty are acute care specialists. The idea of embracing and incorporating geriatric nursing and the nursing home in the curriculum challenges basic values.

Each demonstration site has pursued faculty development activities somewhat differently. Gerontologic and long-term care nursing specialists from nearby universities have been brought to the faculty as consultants. Faculty have attended workshops and conferences, and in most sites several faculty members have attended classes and taken exams leading to certification in gerontologic nursing. Faculty have spent time in nursing homes; in some sites, faculty have taken summer employment in a nursing home. Very successful seminars on gerontologic nursing topics have been developed and offered that were attended by both nursing faculty and nursing home directors of nursing and staff developers. There are rich serendipitous benefits of faculty and nursing home nurses as learner-peers in a seminar.

The faculty development experiences have taught us two important principles: (1) gerontologic/geriatric nursing becomes more interesting to faculty when they know more about it, and (2) even the nursing home becomes more interesting to faculty as familiarity increases.

2. Curriculum change. In all project schools, the curriculum time devoted to geriatric long-term care theory and practice has been increased, content has been improved in terms of recency and sophistication, and clinical education has been vitalized. We have learned a great deal about what to teach, when to teach it, and where to teach it. We hope to share these ideas and experiences through future publication of a curriculum handbook; for now, our earliest work is described in an NLN publication entitled *Associated Degree Nursing and the Nursing Home*, a set of conference papers. One insight worthy of mention: We began with a specific objective to change student attitudes, and our own work along with that of others who have published in the past 2 years suggests to us that we will focus instead on competence. Attitude changes follow the development of competence, we believe.

3. Staff development in the nursing home. Activities to develop nursing home personnel and establish an effective environment for clinical education have taken us on previously untraveled paths, and have been rich with surprises, successes, and disappointments. Nursing education and the nursing home have been strangers, each viewing the other with mistrust and misunderstanding. Staff development for nursing home personnel has taken many forms, including, to list a few examples, special classes and conferences for certified nursing assistants held on campus or televised to local nursing homes, management seminars for directors of nursing, workshops to teach physical assessment skills to staff developers, and the enrollment of nursing home licensed vocational nurses (LVNs) in the ADN program. Partnership activities between the associate degree nursing program and community nursing homes have, in instance after instance, been the match causing kindling already there to burst into flame. A vigorous interfacility ethics committee to respond to the needs of four neighboring nursing homes is one example.

4. Expanding the involvement of the community college as an institution in local concerns regarding health care for the elderly. Not a primary focus, this object has nonetheless led to new networks and programs on all campuses. We are now engaging many of those new networks as we seek to institutionalize project successes to ensure their continued existence after funding is over in 1990.

Use of the nursing home as a clinical education facility for students has figured specifically in the project from the beginning. Our reasoning initially had to do with an explicit purpose to prepare graduates to take entry-level positions in nursing homes as well as in acute care hospitals. Some project schools had no affiliations with nursing homes when we began; others were using the nursing home for clinical placement during a fundamentals course, to learn basic body care skills. We went into the project intending to develop clinical placements late in the students' program for practice of nursing at a more complex level, approaching the role of the registered nurse in the nursing home in ensuring quality of care. We have done that, putting new courses in place, or revising existing ones in the final year of the program.

Looking more broadly at the nursing role in the nursing home has been a learning experience for us all. A new reason for incorporating the nursing home in the clinical education of students has emerged and been articulated by Elaine Tagliareni at Community College of Philadelphia. It is that the acute hospital at the end of the 1980s is a deprived learning environment for basic students. The volatile patient problems, the length of stay, and the wraparound technology inhibit teaching and learning for novices. The nursing home, on the other hand, which begins to look like the acute hospital of the 1970s, is a potentially fruitful learning environment.

Another thing we have found: As the faculty takes on the challenge of increasing the program's sensitivity to the aging of the patient population, curriculum changes are made in every course. Gerontologic content becomes comfortably part of fundamentals, medical-surgical, psychology—even maternal-child nursing with the addition of attention to grandparenting.

Affiliations with nursing homes for clinical education require time to establish. The ingredients of a successful partnership are as follows:

1. Both the nursing program and the nursing home want an

educational affiliation.

2. They develop a trusting relationship with one another.

3. There is communication about the partnership at all levels in the nursing home and the nursing program.

4. Each is willing to change some practices or expectations and to struggle to work out the difficulties.

Nursing homes have commonly never had an academic affiliation; they have much to learn about education of nurses in today's world. Nursing faculties, on the other hand, can carry the devaluing and wrongheaded stereotype too frequently applied to the nursing home and the people who work there: dreadful care delivered by the otherwise unemployable.

These barriers, formidable as they are, can be transformed. Nurse educators have every reason to break down the barriers and create changes in our curriculums. We need to develop relationships with nursing homes that, like our relationships with acute care facilities, enable the placement of students in an effective learning environment. We have a responsibility to prepare today's students for the nursing work of the future.

REFERENCES

National Center for Health Statistics. (1987). *Health statistics on older persons, U.S.* Vital and Health Statistics, Series 3, No. 25. (PHS Publication No. 87-1409). Washington, DC: U.S. Government Printing Office.

National League for Nursing. (1988). *Nursing Student Census with Policy Implications, 1988.* New York: National League for Nursing.

12

LONG-TERM CARE INNOVATIONS: THE ROBERT WOOD JOHNSON TEACHING NURSING HOME PROGRAM

Joyce Colling, PhD, RN
Professor
School of Nursing
Oregon Health Sciences University
Portland, Oregon

There have been several teaching or academic nursing home models developed in recent years from various grants and programs in the United States. The National Institute of Aging has sponsored eight projects with a particular emphasis on research and specifying that a medical school must be involved in the project. Further, these projects state that the research must be biomedical in nature rather than behavioral. The Veterans Administration has also initiated academic nursing homes in some of their 116 long-term care facilities. All of these projects are associated with acute care hospitals in the Veterans Administration system. In addition, the Kellogg Foundation has funded a number of teaching nursing home initiatives with community college nursing programs.

The Robert Wood Johnson (RWJ) Teaching Home initiative was unique because it specified affiliations between university schools of nursing and community nursing homes. The overall goal of the initiative was to promote excellence in nursing care through collaboration with schools of nursing and nursing homes. Two priorities were specified in the grant guidelines. One was to demonstrate qualitative improvement in the standard of nursing care in the affiliating nursing homes. The second was to enhance the movement of patients from acute care hospitals to skilled nursing facilities and to community based care.

There were 11 university schools of nursing and their affiliated nursing homes in the 6-year project which began in 1982. These sites were chosen from a group of more than 100 who initially expressed interest and from 53 institutions who wrote grant applications in response to the foundation's special initiative. The sites selected were:

Rutgers University – Bergen Pines County Hospital

Catholic University – Carroll Manor Nursing Home

Case Western Reserve – Margaret Wagner House

University of Cincinnati – Maple Knoll Village

University of Wisconsin, Madison – Methodist Health Center

Creighton University – Mercy Care and Madonna Centers

University of Utah – Hillhaven Convalescent Center

Oregon Health Sciences University – Benedictine Nursing Center

State University of New York/Binghamton – Willow Point Nursing Home

Georgetown University – Greater S.W. Community Center for Aging

Rush-Presbyterian – Edward Hines Jr. Veterans Administration Extended Care Center

Each of these sites built from existing strengths and, while the general goals of the program were the same for all sites, each university and nursing home affiliation developed specific objectives on which to focus during the project.

THE OREGON PROJECT

In Oregon, the Benedictine Nursing Center (BNC) had long been known for its holistic approach to care of the elderly across multiple settings and its innovative approaches to care of the elderly. It has served as a clinical facility for nursing and allied health programs for many years but not with the University School of Nursing. In addition, it pioneered in employing a master's prepared nurse clinician in mental health to address the special needs of elderly residents. Out of a commitment to the dignity of every human person, it has maintained a favorable ratio of professional and nonprofessional nursing staff to patients and has developed a strong nursing leadership component. The management of the center is based on a philosophy of mutual trust and shared decision making. Consequently, it provided an excellent clinical site for the development of future practitioners and the generation of knowledge throughout the Teaching Nursing Home (TNH) Project.

The Oregon Health Sciences University, School of Nursing also drew on several strengths. It had a strong tradition of practice-centered research and it expected faculty to maintain expertise in a special area of nursing through continuing links with clinical practice areas. In addition, the school also contains several senior faculty with advanced preparation in gerontological nursing as well as a growing recognition of the need to prepare more nurses to provide for the special care needs of the elderly. At the school, the TNH project acted as catalyst to stimulate the inclusion of additional content and clinical practice in geriatric care in the curriculum and clinical research focused on care of the elderly.

Program Goals and Commitment

The overall goals of the TNH in Oregon were to: (1) promote excellence in the care of geriatric clients through clinical research; (2) provide educational opportunities for students in nursing and other disciplines; and (3) model innovations in the care of geriatric clients for the larger nursing community. Each year of the project, specific objectives were identified under each of these broad goals.

Strong administrative commitment in both institutions remained consistent throughout the project; however, the primary goals of the institutions were different and a number of specific issues had to be resolved for the TNH project to achieve the rather ambitious goals that had been identified. Some of these difficult questions were: How could two institutions influence the perceptions of the other regarding care of the elderly? how could the balance of power and control be established and maintained when one institution held the purse strings? and how could collaborative relationships be established and maintained when the benefits of the relationship were not clear to either institution? Early in the project, a consultant in organizational development was hired to assist in resolving some of these issues. A major outcome of this process was a TNH Mission Statement which provided clarification and identity for the TNH (see Figure 1). In addition, it was determined that the TNH was to be a separate entity created to achieve goals compatible with, but separate from either sponsoring institution. These activities were major turning points in the project's development and progress, and provided the framework against which the TNH staff could work through problems and achieve its goals.

Immediate Outcomes

The outcomes of the TNH project in Oregon are organized around four areas. First, it has established a teaching model using master's prepared clinical specialists in gerontology who provide direct care and consultation in the nursing home as well as supervise nursing students who come to the nursing home for a portion of their clinical practice. There are now two clinical specialists who have joint appointments with the School of Nursing and the BNC. They are based at the BNC and only travel to the university when specified in their job descriptions. This has made it possible for over 100 undergraduate and a number of graduate students to gain experience in gerontological nursing at the BNC, where 6 years ago only a few students had this type of experience at any facility. These two faculty have also made significant contributions to the School of Nursing regarding curriculum matters and have added further emphasis to the need for increased experiences in geriatric care. These efforts have made it possible to establish a separate required undergraduate course in gerontological nursing at the School of Nursing.

A second major outcome from the TNH project has been clinical research. Several projects were completed focusing on significant clinical problems in long-term care. The value of this research is that it was generated from clinical practice issues of concern in the nursing home and in turn can directly effect their practice of nursing. Some examples are: an evaluation of the effectiveness of an exercise and relaxation program to decrease agitation among Alzheimer patients; a 2-year qualitative study to identify staff behaviors which families of dying patients found most helpful; a study to develop an effective management program for certain patients with urinary incontinence; the development and evaluation of an outreach program for families caring for a demented family member; and a study to identify types of wandering behavior and determine appropriate nursing interventions.

The third outcome focuses on increased opportunities for nursing staff at the BNC to obtain further education or share innovations in care with other health care professionals. For instance, one primary nurse published an article on the management of skin tears while several others presented clinical innovations at a TNH conference.

Fourth, the TNH has been able to provide start-up resources for other projects, such as a feasibility study to determine the need for a BNC-based home health agency, and preliminary assistance that resulted in federal funding for a major research grant to treat urinary incontinence as well as a federal training grant to train mental health specialists in geriatric nursing care.

Long-Term Outcomes

Nationally, the 11 RWJ Teaching Nursing Home project sites have stimulated considerable knowledge about enhancing the quality of care for elderly nursing home clients and in developing a variety of affiliative relationships between schools of nursing and long-term care facilities. Each of the sites has some unique aspects, but there has been a profound impact on all of the staff associated with the projects. Hundreds of nursing students as well as other health care students have benefited from the project, as have the nursing faculties and nursing home staffs. While the external evaluation of the program is not yet public, there are strong indications that the two priorities specified in the RWJ initiative have been achieved and that collaboration between nursing homes and schools of nursing have enhanced the care of elderly clients significantly.

For us in Oregon, the TNH project has provided the stimulus to combine the expertise of two strong institutions to achieve objectives which neither could have reached independently. Further, it has served to lower the barriers between academia and service settings, to help find answers to the many clinical problems which nursing faces, has offered nursing home nurses additional educational opportunities, and has provided many student nurses with special clinical skills to care for elderly clients. Finally, it has provided a springboard for continuing collaboration through the BNC Long-Term Institute, enabling the school and the nursing center to continue to expand their collaborative efforts on behalf of elderly clients.

FIGURE 1. Mission Statement for Oregon Teaching Nursing Home Program

The Teaching Nursing Home Program (TNH) is a joint venture of the Oregon Health Sciences University School of Nursing (OHSU/SON) and the Benedictine Nursing Center (BNC) for the purpose of enriching both the patient care of the Benedictine Nursing Center and the education of nursing students of OHSU/SON. The TNH is dependent for its existence on both the OHSU/SON and the BNC, but it is a separate entity with its own mission. Its focus is education and research in clinical practice in long-term care; specifically at the BNC.

We believe that patient care will be enriched by more conscious practice of theory and research based nursing. Careful scientific testing and articulation of specific approaches to problems of care of the elderly and chronically ill will improve and enhance care of the patients at the BNC. Dissemination of knowledge gained will provide guidance for enhanced care of patients in other settings.

We believe that education of nursing students will be enriched by the experience in the long-term care setting, with creative practitioners as role models and mentors.

We believe that both patient care and education will be enhanced by mutual exchange between nurses and faculty of OHSU/SON and nurses of staff at BNC, by faculty practicing and/or teaching in the clinical setting, and staff of BNC teaching classes at the School of Nursing. Faculty and staff will learn from one another.

The role of the TNH is that of a catalyst for change for both OHSU/SON and BNC, with no direct authority to change either. Its function is to stimulate more effective interventions with patients and with students. It will raise issues and suggest program directions to both OHSU/SON and BNC. It may also provide both institutions with the personnel, resources, and/or linkages to carry out projects that relate to the focus of the TNH, i.e., research and education on aspects of nursing care of the long-term patient.

Because its focus is on study and articulation of patient care issues tested in a clinical setting, it will also be concerned and involved in action relating to public policy, systems of care reimbursement, advocacy, and especially the role of nursing in the care of the chronically ill and elderly. While firmly based in the field of nursing, the TNH will be committed to a holistic approach and the interdisciplinary process in the delivery of care to the long-term care population.

13

THE VALUE OF THE TEACHING NURSING HOME AFFILIATION FROM A FACILITY PERSPECTIVE

Sister Lucia Gamroth, MS, MPA, RN
Associate Administrator
Benedictine Nursing Center
Mt. Angel, Oregon

WHY SUCH A VENTURE?

Facilities saw this as an opportunity to introduce students to the world of professional nursing in long-term care (LTC). Nursing in LTC is different from nursing in other settings. The complexity of the problems that the frail, often chronically ill elderly present is very challenging and nurses in long-term care have discovered things that work for patients.

The world of LTC is complex, not just from a clinical point of view, but as a political, socio-economic system. Advocates for improved quality of care push for reform while at the same time crying about the expense of nursing home care. Since diagnosis related groups (DRGs) have been implemented in hospitals, nursing homes are caring for very ill persons for a small percentage of the cost of a hospital day, while nursing home reimbursement structures remain rigid.

Facilities saw this as an opportunity to ground the education of student nurses, undergraduate and graduate, in some of these realities. They saw it as an opportunity to change the image of LTC that many students and faculty hold about nursing homes as undesirable places to be or to work.

What about the education of the practitioners who are currently practicing in long-term care? There is a growing body of research and theory that is directly related to nursing practice in long-term care: decubitus care, pain management, the use of restraints, management of wandering behavior. Practitioners need to be aware of current research findings that can improve their clinical practice and to contribute their expertise to that body of knowledge.

Improved education and improved practice are the reasons why all of us entered into the Teaching Nursing Home (TNH) projects. The sections that follow describe and highlight the process used to reach several of the goals we established.

Educational Opportunities

A number of strategies were employed to stimulate nursing faculty and nursing staff to contribute to the achievement of the goal of increasing educational opportunities for students and nursing staff. First, a TNH open house at the Benedictine Nursing Center (BNC) was scheduled as a part of faculty orientation in the fall. Tours of the facility were conducted and posters of regular center-sponsored as well as TNH-sponsored programs and projects were displayed. A brochure was developed identifying potential clinical research projects for students and/or faculty as well as outlining potential clinical opportunities for students.

Secondly, a yearly spring TNH colloquium was begun which has provided a forum for TNH staff, graduate students, and BNC nurses to share the results of clinical projects or innovations in geriatric nursing care with each other and the nursing faculty and staff. The site was alternated each year, which provided a mechanism to introduce BNC staff to the university campus, encourage more faculty to visit the BNC, and stimulated dialogue among faculty, staff, and students.

A third strategy employed to increase mutual awareness of university and nursing center opportunities was the establishment of joint appointments of two gerontological nursing clinical specialists. Their presence and influence in their respective departments as expert clinicians and competent faculty members have been vital in furthering this major goal.

The TNH provided educational opportunities for a number of nurses at the BNC by sending them to workshops, bringing various experts to the BNC for presentation, and offering one course at the BNC. It provided partial funding for advanced degrees for two nurses and a BSN for a third.

Clinical Research

Nurses in the practice arena have been critical of the lack of applicability of nursing research to clinical practice issues. This need and concern were addressed in the TNH by involving all TNH staff in the generation of a list of practice issues of highest concern to the RNs. The issues were evaluated for relevance, then prioritized and developed into researchable questions. A number of approaches were used to examine the research questions, which served to introduce staff to the use of differing methodologies as well as to enhance understanding of the link between research and practice.

The TNH staff also decided that a formal procedure to screen research proposals was needed. A group was formed, composed of BNC staff, TNH staff, a methodologist from the School of Nursing, and a member of the BNC board, to establish review guidelines and to serve as a review committee. The responsibilities of the review committee were to determine the merits and appropriateness of proposals, protect patient rights, and prevent overburdening of staff.

Delivery System

Two changes in the delivery system, as a result of grant support, were the implementation of primary nursing and the development of a home health agency. The primary nursing model is organized so each primary nurse (two on each unit) has 24-hour responsibility for care for the duration of the patient's stay at the facility. The two clinical specialists act as consultants to the primary nurses, hence they have a ready, knowledgeable resource on which to draw when a difficult care problem arises.

Based upon a feasibility study conducted with grant support, the BNC expanded its personal care service in the community to a full service home health agency that provides a continuum of care for those discharged from the facility or for those not needing inpatient services.

COSTS

What does it cost for a facility to enter into the world of education? There are material costs of space for students and research, lockers, added telephone and correspondence, parking, and additional laundry. Those costs are fairly easily documented. There are personnel costs such as primary nursing differentials and clinical specialist positions that are also easily documented. There are other costs that are not so obvious: the human resources of time, energy, and commitment that it takes to succeed at this venture. There is the psychic cost "of one more thing." The requests of the professional community about the TNH affiliation involve telephone calls, photocopying of materials, visits, consultation, and orchestration of meetings, which is all very time consuming.

Preliminary results of the external evaluation program indicate that the overall project was successful in preventing hospitalizations and clinical problems such as decubiti. What about the costs of prevention or the added costs of treating the patient in the facility rather than transferring him or her to the hospital? Have those costs been recognized and accounted for in such a manner that the facility can document and be reimbursed for the cost of prevention? While administrators agree that there are added costs for educational programs of this type, little has been done to research and document the costs. Further research is needed to answer the cost questions.

The TNH project is not like starting a home health agency that is an extension of your current program under your philosophy, goals, and management. The TNH is a matter of blending two institutions with different purposes, different structures, different expectations, and different economic constraints. The investment is extensive and the benefits are many.

BENEFITS

What did administrators perceive as the real benefits of this program? Attitudinal changes by School of Nursing faculty have resulted in new course content focused on gerontological nursing, more faculty interested in research about older adults, and a greater appreciation of the professional nurse in the LTC setting and the complex needs of the elderly. Many students have been exposed to long-term care as a part of their training. And we are beginning to see those graduates select LTC as the preferred practice setting.

Facility staff have become more systematic in identifying clinical problems, have increased their use of literature sources, and initiated clinical research. Numbers of staff have received advanced education or ANA certification as gerontological nurses. Clinical staff have developed a spirit of inquiry and are considered to be on the cutting edge of gerontological nursing practice. Program changes, such as mobility programs and primary nursing programs, have been incorporated as a result of the project.

Multiple products such as articles, book chapters, and videos have resulted from these projects. All of these are efforts to disseminate current knowledge and experience in clinical areas of the TNH models.

The new affiliations between schools of nursing and nursing homes have a credibility in the world of research and public policy. They speak with authority on issues of LTC reform and professional nursing in LTC. They attract additional research and education grants as a result of the affiliation between the clinical and university site.

Perhaps the greatest testimony to the success of this effort is the number of TNH affiliations that are continuing into the future. For the Oregon site, one of the most exciting outcomes of the TNH was the formation of the Benedictine Institute for Long-Term Care. The purpose of the Institute is to pioneer new approaches in research and education and to generate and disseminate new knowledge concerning the long-term care of older persons.

> The Benedictine Institute program is, in many ways, an extension of the TNH; however, it will expand and broaden the TNH goals to influence the entire long-term care system in Oregon and the region. Institute programs will, therefore, be directed at a wide range of people, including consumers, health care professionals, family caregivers, and health care policymakers. A major focus will be on providing educational and training programs to meet needs that are currently not being met. Developing effective clinical methods in long term- care and sharing those with care providers will also be a top priority.

> The past five years have been marked by growth, change, frustration, and a continuing commitment to provide high quality care to the frail elderly by all the TNH staff. The project has acted as a powerful stimulus to find better ways to achieve this commitment. The formation of a unique Institute holds the promise of continuing the commitment through long term collaborative relationships between an educational and a service institution. (Colling & Gamroth, 1988, p. 1986)

REFERENCES

Colling, J., & Gamroth, L. (1988). Oregon Health Sciences University School of Nursing and the Benedictine Nursing Center. In N.R. Small & M.B. Walsh (Eds.), *Teaching nursing homes: The nursing perspective*. Owings Mills, MD: National Health Publishing.

Testing and Accreditation

14

LIFTING THE VEIL OF SECRECY

Maria K. Mitchell, MS, RN
Senior Vice President
Community Health Accreditation Program
New York, New York

It seems remarkable that it is nearly the year 2000, and we are living in a society that is feeding information to China, a country thousands of miles away, via fax machine, to keep the fires of revolution burning, all in the name of democracy. Yet, we are gathered here to debate the appropriateness of giving United States citizens adequate information to make decisions about where to receive their health care.

Perhaps, rather than "Lifting the Veil of Secrecy," this could more appropriately be titled, "Lifting the Iron Curtain of Secrecy."

It seems unthinkable that providers of health care, education, or any service to the public would not yet understand that the consumer has a right to information. More importantly, the only real way to achieve quality is to provide meaningful information to the public. But, as a society, we have a long way to go.

Why is it that providers are so reluctant to share information with the public? Information that will let their customers know how they measure up to quality standards? I think it is fair to say that most providers believe they are doing a quality job. So is this "veil of secrecy" then simply a societal mindset established early on in the area of accreditation?

On October 12, 1988, *The Wall Street Journal* ran a front-page story on hospital accreditation and how it is not serving the public. The article discussed the history of hospital accreditation and described its roots as follows:

A policy of keeping hospital deficiencies under tight wraps reflects the
spirit of cooperation. The Joint Commission has kept the findings of its
hospital surveys confidential since the group was established by the
American College of Surgeons in 1951. (The College had conducted the
first nationwide hospital inspection in 1919—and after reviewing the
dismal findings at a meeting at the Waldorf-Astoria Hotel in New York, it
tossed them into the hotel's furnace). Without the promise of confidentiality, the Joint Commission argues, hospitals wouldn't voluntarily agree to
open their private records to outsiders.

It is ironic, but the very fact that this article made public the issue of
disclosure, and let consumers know that such important information
was being withheld has, in the last 6 months, caused the *first* amendment to the Joint Commission's disclosure policy in over 30 years.

As a result of the tremendous public outcry caused by *The Wall Street
Journal* article, the Joint Commission recently approved a plan to
provide selected survey data to the Health Care Financing Administration (HCFA) only. It is HCFA that may choose to make the information
public. The Joint Commission itself will only make public the names of
conditionally accredited hospitals.

As evidenced by the public outcry caused by *The Wall Street Journal*
article, the public has come to understand that they are being short-
changed. Consumers and purchasers of health care products and
services know that there are good providers and some not so good
providers.

They are tired of finding out, by receiving and paying for less than
adequate treatment, who the bad providers are. Consumers and their
agents who pay for a big percentage of the care—insurers and business—are determined to find a meaningful way to choose the good
providers.

Of course, at the heart of disclosure, is quality and the search for
quality health care services. People are tired of receiving and paying for
poor quality health care services. And, as happened with the American
automobile industry, consumers are beginning to revolt because they
are not satisfied. We witnessed the power of consumer demand for
quality in the near demise of the American automobile industry. We can
be sure that the people of this nation are no more sanguine about their
own health than they were about their cars, particularly since they are
paying more out of their pockets for health care.

A 1989 Harvard/Harris poll compared the Canadian and American
health care systems and found that over 50 percent of Canadians, who
have free access to their health care system, were satisfied with their
health care system. Conversely, over 89 percent of Americans were
dissatisfied with the health care in this country. That means that only
10 percent of the people in the United States may be satisfied with the
health care delivery system in this country. A terrible report card.

The issue of providing good quality care cannot, of course, be divorced from the issue of how quality itself is defined. It has been argued that even the most technically sophisticated measures of outcome are never going to speak for themselves without ambiguity and without debate. The very notion of quality is contestable because it is liable to change over time and is culture specific. More importantly, most desirable outcomes are continuing processes, especially for people with terminal illnesses. For those people, the way they are treated—with kindness, sensitivity, etc.—is always most important. And who but the recipient of care has the right to judge that?

The central issue then becomes that a quality revolution should be unequivocally and primarily focused on consumers of care and should be predicated on providing consumers with information identified to be most important (by consumers themselves as well as providers) concerning decisions about quality.

In the hospitals, that means nosocomial infection rates, rates of recidivism, and rates of postoperative complications. In home care, that means how long on average it takes to clear decubitus ulcers, rehospitalization data, and so forth.

Consumers' perceptions of quality affect their choice among health care alternatives. For competitive markets to work most efficiently and effectively, relevant consumer information about quality is of vital importance to allow consumers to choose the superior provider among competitive alternatives. Otherwise, there is an inherent conflict of interest in making determinations about the best quality providers.

Even though consumer conceptions of quality often tend to be dismissed as highly "personal," making a patient feel secure and comforted as well as able to understand the treatment regimen may well be important factors in the success of the patient's treatment program and ultimate recovery. Studies have demonstrated that consumers want more information about their plans of care and more involvement in developing their own plans of care.

In any future major reform of national health policies, consumers should be integrally involved in defining quality in its various dimensions and aspects. They should be given vital information regarding quality and encouraged to make choices related to quality health care. Public and private agencies in charge of quality review, including accrediting bodies, should be required to adopt public disclosure policies that would provide consumers with important information related to quality, as an important first step.

There is no better way to assure quality than to let the purchasers of care hold the providers publicly accountable for the services they provide. I think if this happened in every sector of our delivery system we would see fewer but more effective providers and, more importantly, a healthier nation.

At CHAP (Community Health Accreditation Program), we have adopted a policy of full public disclosure because a definition of quality that doesn't consider the consumer, or a standard that doesn't hold up under public scrutiny, is no measure of quality. I hope that this is the beginning of a trend in health care.

I could not help but think of the difference between CHAP and other health care accrediting bodies last week when reading an article in the *New York Times*. In discussing George Bush's long-awaited emergence as something of a leader during the European NATO talks, it said that perhaps Mr. Bush would finally now find out that it is far more exciting to be an agent of change, and that it is far more challenging and rewarding to be an innovator, than a keeper of the status quo.

Ronald Reagan's defense policies were appropriate for the time, but trying to maintain that status quo and ignoring the people's desire for change did great damage to the public's view of George Bush as a leader. In finally recognizing the need to change with the times and acting on it, he emerged a hero.

Perhaps the medically dominated health care system will look to CHAP and learn the same lesson—for the public's sake.

REFERENCES

Bogdenich, W. (1988, October 12). Prized by hospitals, accreditation hides perils patients face. *The Wall Street Journal*, p. 1.

15

PUBLIC DISCLOSURE: LIFTING THE VEIL OF SECRECY ON ACCREDITATION

Howard L. Simmons, PhD
Executive Director
Middle States Commission on Higher Education
Philadelphia, Pennsylvania

It must be recognized at the outset that any discussion of public disclosure is practically impossible without corresponding reference to confidentiality as an essential ingredient in the accrediting process. As the Council on Postsecondary Accreditation (COPA) points out in its *Policy Statement on Disclosure, Confidentiality and Integrity of the Accrediting Process*:

> Concern for the integrity and effectiveness of the investigative and deliberative process involves *respect for confidentiality of information* required and evaluated. The purposes are endangered and the process is weakened when disclosure of aspects of the process inhibits both the institution's or program's ability to provide complete information and assess itself candidly and the accrediting bodies' ability to render sound judgements. The relationship between the accrediting body and the institution or program is private and voluntary. Accrediting decisions are, however, used as a consideration in many formal actions by different publics—government funding agencies, scholarship commissions, foundations, employers, counselors, and potential students. Accrediting bodies have thus come to be viewed as quasi-public entities operating "for the common good" or "in the public interest" with certain responsibilities to the many groups which interact with the educational community. Thus the legitimate needs of

accrediting bodies or those of their members for maintaining and preserv-
ing the integrity of the process must be reconciled with broader societal
needs requiring disclosure of basic and essential information. (COPA,
October 1984, p. 1)

When public disclosure is juxtaposed with confidentiality, we are
presented with a great dilemma and a need to maintain in perfect
balance the often conflicting requirements of the two concepts. Therefore, it is necessary to address both public disclosure *and* confidentiality
in order to achieve a better understanding about what can and should
be done about these two important issues in the accreditation process.

The title of this paper, "Lifting the Veil of Secrecy," conjures up
images of intrigue. How could such an improbable metaphor apply to
accreditation or the process of decision making in accreditation when
there is such a wide network of persons involved in the peer review
process? How could there possibly be a "veil of secrecy" when educators
in general don't know how to keep secrets? To be sure, we have not
always been clear about what accreditation is, what accreditation can
do, what accreditation cannot do, what accreditation decisions really
mean, why accreditation is really important, who are the consumers of
accreditation, and what the various publics should know about accreditation. But this can hardly be called a "veil of secrecy."

Although it would be naive to believe that we would no longer have
an issue of public disclosure and confidentiality if everyone had a
perfect understanding of and appreciation for the accreditation process
as it is practiced in the United States, I do believe that if that were the
situation the topic would be much easier to address. How do we achieve
such understanding, especially on the part of accreditation's different
publics?

One of the clues to increased public understanding can be found in
the brief description in the preliminary program announcing the 1989
NLN Convention: "The public's right to expect quality from accredited
institutions includes the public's right to know about services in
language that is accessible, accurate, and illuminating." Particular
emphasis should be placed on the portion of that statement which
reads, *"in language that is accessible, accurate, and illuminating."*

One serious problem is the lack of suitably prepared and packaged
information about what the accreditation process is, what it can do, and
what it cannot do. And, yes, that information should be in a language
that can be understood by persons other than those who earn their
livelihoods administering regional, institutional, and program accreditation protocols.

Lack of understanding of the accrediting process is not confined to
what one might call the general public, since there are many faculty
members, administrators, and members of governing boards who have

little or no understanding of the nature and impact of either institutional or programmatic accreditation.

Just as textbooks in certain disciplines appear often to be written more for the faculty than the students, so it is that accreditation manuals containing standards, procedures, guidelines, and the like are written by and for those most closely involved in staff or committee work. Even though most of the literature on accreditation prepared by regional, institutional, and specialized bodies is tastefully done and generally responds to the need of constituents' members, the literature is not always that appealing to most members of the public-at-large. This is precisely because the style, format, language, and content have not in most cases been designed or selected with the public consumer in mind.

Would it be unthinkable to suggest that accrediting bodies might improve the appeal of their publications by enlisting the aid of a marketing consultant? In almost any other field of endeavor every attempt is made to get a product or service better known, understood, and used. Appropriate packaging is the key not only to getting the general public to be more aware of the product or service but also to help avoid misunderstandings about what the product or service can and cannot do.

In the field of accreditation, it might even be helpful to have a book like "All You Ever Wanted to Know About Accreditation But Were Afraid to Ask." The bottom line is, can't the basic information about accreditation be presented in a more interesting, informative, and lively format? Don't we have the wherewithal to design colorful and informative brochures that contain frequently asked questions about the nature and workings of the accreditation process? Examples: Is accreditation like the "Good Housekeeping" seal of approval? Does accreditation mean that my courses are certified? Does it mean that I can automatically transfer all of my credits? When you accredit, aren't you really concerned about the quality and reputation of the faculty? When you accredit, what ratings or rankings do you give the colleges? (No! Accreditation is not like *U.S. News and World Report!*) What are the ten best programs (or institutions) that you accredit? Do you ever *disaccredit* any institution? If so, from how many did you remove accreditation in the last five years?

The list could go on and on. But one thing is clear: There are answers to these questions even though the answers are not always simple. Even more significant is that we usually respond with too much jargon and ambiguity. And at least some of the time we're giving only partial answers because of our commitment to confidentiality or our policy of limited disclosure or both. As a result, we may be withholding important information that consumers (e.g., students, parents, legislators) need for informed choices. The question is, can we be more straightforward about the actions taken with respect to an institution's or program's accreditation without compromising or jeopardizing that institution's or program's standing?

While we must still develop more appealing and informative material about accreditation for the general consumer, we must also reconsider some of the sacred cows about confidentiality and disclosure. It is only fair to say that some accrediting bodies have already made great strides in expanding information that is disclosed to the public concerning accreditation actions. As F. Taylor Jones, the first executive director of the Middle States Commission on Higher Education, said more than 30 years ago, "We must do more than reveal the accreditation status of the institution."

Although most who have studied these issues or have adopted more liberal policies concerning public disclosure would agree that certain aspects of the accreditation process must be kept confidential, there is room for greater disclosure without compromising the process. We can all agree that the hundreds of thousands of volunteer peer reviewers must be able to continue their evaluation activities without fear of intimidation or reprisal; institutional constituent groups must be able to continue the process of assessing institutional effectiveness without undue political interference or pressure; accrediting committees and commissions must be able to continue discussing and making decisions about the accreditation of institutions in a manner that protects all parties and the integrity of the process itself; and in general the accrediting body must keep inviolate the confidential nature of the information it receives.

However, that does not mean that everything that happens in the accrediting process is confidential or has a veil of secrecy. Naturally, should accrediting bodies act in this manner, there would be perhaps a perception among the general public that accrediting activities are star chamber proceedings that involve a chosen few. The reality—though not always apparent to those not directly involved in the accrediting process—is that there is a great deal of openness and trust among site visitors and institutional hosts, precisely because the evaluation process itself is confidential. There is a certain level of comfort that is mutually shared with colleagues as peers that sensitive information will not be divulged to "outsiders." Thus, it is commonly understood that the documents (i.e., self-studies, evaluation reports, official action letters) and the process (evaluation visit, self-assessment, deliberations by accrediting body) must be protected by policies of confidentiality. None of this means, however, that all aspects of the accrediting process are confidential or shrouded in a veil of secrecy.

Louis H. Heilbron, in an important monograph in the late 1970s on the subject of confidentiality and accreditation, probably summed up the issue best when he concluded:

> The principle of preserving a measure of confidentiality in order to enable
> an agency to function . . . when applied to accrediting agencies . . . appears
> to be more a matter of public policy, to be urged upon legislators consid-
> ering restrictive legislation against agency operations and upon courts
> considering sweeping demands to compel disclosure of information that
> leads to the improvement of educational standards—information that
> would not have been given except under conditions of confidentiality.
> (Heilbron, 1976, p. 28)

Heilbron is right on target when he recommends that "accrediting agencies should restudy their procedures (with respect to records and meetings) to be certain that they are as open to public scrutiny as the essential purposes of accreditation permit" (Heilbron, 1976, p. 29).

Can we be more straightforward about the actions taken with respect to an institution's or program's accreditation? This brings us to the other essential part of our topic—disclosure. After an accrediting body has defined what information about an institution will be kept confidential, it must determine what will be made available to the public and should specify to whom and when disclosure is to be made. It should also indicate in what form the information will be made available.

In addition and especially in view of the newly revised US Department of Education accrediting agency recognition criteria that require *all* accreditation actions to be reported to the Secretary of Education, both the accrediting agency and the institution must be clear about respective responsibilities for disclosing negative accreditation actions. To be sure, this change in recognition criteria may indeed have the effect of accelerating the process of broadening disclosure of accrediting information to the public.

Therefore, when disclosure is broadened to include a wider public, appropriate consideration must be given to adequate due process procedures, so that the interests and rights of all parties are protected. That is precisely the reason why the procedures for disclosure are important, since the premature release of negative information could do irreparable harm to the institution, currently enrolled students, prospective students, the accrediting body itself, and the public-at-large. Significant damage could be done even though, ostensibly, the disclosure of the "negative" information was to protect the public interest.

That is why I would argue that all accreditation actions should be disclosed to the general public only after an institution or program has exhausted all appeals. The primary difficulty with this stance is that a worst-case scenario where the interests of the public might be violated could warrant the prior release of such information. But this is only one form of disclosure. Others might include:

- The development of policy statements on fair practice

- The implementation of a series of public meetings by the accrediting commissions for the purpose of discussing policy issues

- The use of press conferences, television spots, and news releases about significant policy development with respect to accreditation

- The use of eye-appealing information brochures as well as videotapes and other audiovisual materials about the "nuts and bolts" of accreditation

- The joint development and use of statements of affiliation status about an institution or program that could be made available to the public upon request

- The inclusion of larger numbers of public representatives in the accrediting process (i.e., in on-site visit teams, commissions, or committees)

- The development and use of a more effective statement of ethics for institutions/programs, evaluators, consultants, and agency staff regarding confidentiality and disclosure

Whether regional, institutional, or specialized bodies have adopted or plan to adopt some or all of these means to disclose more information to various publics, it is clear that current realities in higher education and in our larger society demand more inclusive policies with respect to accrediting activity, if for no other reason that to gain wider acceptance of and public confidence in the process.

And as COPA admonishes in its statement on *The Judicial and Legislative Context for Disclosure of Accrediting Information:*

> The best protection against judicial interference is constant review of procedures and practices to assure that they are as open to public scrutiny as the continued effectiveness of the process allows, and that there is optimum disclosure of information essential for serving the public interest. (COPA, August 1984, p.1)

Even though the veil of secrecy is much thinner and more vulnerable than the public might surmise, it nonetheless must be lifted. It will probably be illuminating to find that there are no dark, smoke-filled rooms, and that the thousands of "ambassadors of accreditation" really do have quality and excellence as their goal.

REFERENCES

Heilbron, L.H. (1976). Confidentiality and accreditation: An occasional paper. Washington, DC: Council on Postsecondary Accreditation (COPA).

Council on Postsecondary Accreditation (COPA). (1984 August). The judicial and legislative context for disclosure of accrediting information. Washington, DC: Author.

Council on Postsecondary Accreditation (COPA) (1984 October). Policy statement on disclosure, confidentiality and the integrity of the accrediting process. Washington, DC: Author.

16

ANSWERING THE QUESTION OF WHETHER SUCCESS ON THE STATE BOARDS BE CONSIDERED A SIGNIFICANT OUTCOME MEASURE FOR EDUCATIONAL PROGRAMS

Carole A. Anderson, PhD, RN, FAAN
Professor and Dean
College of Nursing
The Ohio State University
Columbus, Ohio

In answer to the question of whether success on the state boards be considered a significant outcome measure for educational programs, my answer is, definitively, no. The strength of my opinion is based on a very simple rationale. Professional nursing education is much more than preparation for a licensure examination. A professional education is theoretically, conceptually, and pragmatically very different from successful completion of the licensing exam. If we design curricula focused on enhancing a student's chances of success on a licensing examination, we will be, in a very real sense, violating the essential purposes of an education.

Licensure has as its fundamental purpose the protection of the public from unqualified practitioners (Kelly, 1981). The authority of the state licensing board is derived from the police power given to each state by the Fourteenth Amendment. Licensure confers the exclusive right to practice, it defines the scope of practice, and it ensures a minimum level of competence designed to protect the public's health and safety (Kelly, 1981).

The 1979 study of credentialing in nursing (ANA, 1979) utilized the following definition of licensure:

> *Licensure*: Licensure is a process by which an agency of state government grants permission to individuals accountable for the practice of a profession to engage in the practice of that profession and prohibits all others from legally doing so. It permits use of a particular title. Its purpose is to protect the public by ensuring a minimum level of professional competence. Established standards and methods of evaluation are used to determine eligibility for initial licensure and for periodic renewal. Effective means are employed for taking action against licensees for acts of professional misconduct, incompetence, and/or negligence.

That definition incorporates the concepts of titling, exclusive right to practice, protection of the public, definition of minimum competence, and the notion that the government agency responsible for licensure is also responsible for establishing standards and methods of evaluation to determine eligibility and also the design and implementation of means for action against acts of individual incompetence, negligence, or professional misconduct.

The history of licensure in nursing parallels the history of licensure in other professions (Kelly, 1981), beginning with an early history lacking both a clear definition of nursing and, most importantly, standards for education. This allowed a variety of differently prepared individuals to call themselves nurses and to engage in the practice of nursing. In response to this lack of quality control, professional organizations such as the National League for Nursing and the American Nurses' Association organized to establish mechanisms that would bring greater congruence to the preparation for professional practice and to the assurance of minimal competency. Mandatory state licensure was the result.

Conceptually and pragmatically, education is very different from licensure. The purpose of education is multifaceted and highly individualized. It is a voluntary, rather than regulatory, activity and is designed to improve the capacity of individuals to contribute to society and hence to the general welfare of its citizens.

The general purposes of higher education are to:

- enable individuals to understand the physical, biological, and social world
- contribute to society through successful role enactment in personal, social, professional, and community roles
- advance the level of societal functioning

Professional nursing education is higher education. Over the past several years, there have been five major studies and reports of our system of higher education, particularly concerning the outcomes of student learning. These blue-ribbon panels have brought severe criticism to bear on contemporary higher education and have urged a return to a more liberal and general education. The overall theme of these published reports is that college and university education has deteriorated into narrowly focused technical education that is oriented more toward job/career than toward broad-based knowledge and understanding of our history, people, and the world in which we live.

Many critics trace the origins of the current situation to the sixties, when the hue-and-cry of student activists was for a relevant education as well as for autonomy in the selection of courses; in other words, for fewer university-mandated requirements. In the ensuing years, making education more relevant amounted to narrowing its focus and targeting it more toward preparation for jobs and careers. Critics such as Alan Bloom, author of *The Closing of the American Mind*, believed that universities and their faculty had given away their prerogatives, indeed, abandoned their moral obligations, when they conceded to students' demands.

As a result of these major studies, many colleges and universities have been undergoing curriculum reform to reinstate general education requirements for all majors that will, they believe, more completely fulfill the goals of liberal education.

The current curriculum reform urges a return to an enhanced general or liberal education with prescribed requirements. The spirit behind this reform is to ensure that the graduates of our colleges and universities are *educated*, not just specifically trained. The Ohio State University is not immune from the current tide. For the past year, a university faculty committee and committees in all the colleges have suggested curriculum reform that is geared toward providing students with a more balanced and well-rounded education. Education should enable all students to obtain the knowledge, attitudes, and skills that will allow them to emerge from the university with an understanding of the past and the present as well as a sense of self that wants both to strive for continued learning and to work with others to facilitate the further development of the human potential.

This model curriculum (Ohio State University, June, 1988), developed in the Colleges of the Arts and Sciences, would be required of all majors. The second phase of the curriculum reform is to mandate that professional programs incorporate this model to the greatest extent possible and also to review the requirements in the majors. The overall goal is to ensure basic competencies across all majors and programs.

I am going to use the model curriculum developed at The Ohio State University as an illustration of contemporary thought regarding the characteristics of an educated person and to expand on the rationale underlying my position on the question posed in this paper.

The OSU curriculum framework incorporates several components:

- Writing and related skills
- Quantitative and logical skills
- Foreign language
- Social diversity in the United States
- Natural science
- Social science
- Arts and humanities

Writing and related skills are the foundation upon which all the others build. These foundation courses enable students to emerge from the university with the ability to write, read, engage in critical thinking, and express themselves verbally. To think that students have graduated from universities without these skills is almost incomprehensible. However, there is ample evidence to suggest that there has been a lack of accountability at all levels of education to ensure the acquisition of increasing competence in these areas. Educators are certainly aware of the diminished ability of our students in terms of these skills. Given the information explosion, it is also true that we probably have paid little attention to further developing these skills in the professional curriculum—we feel we have too much to cover as it is.

The second part of the framework for general education is the development of quantitative and logical skills. Students will complete courses that provide them with the knowledge of how to engage in logical reasoning, do basic mathematical computation, and reach reasonable, logical conclusions by analyzing data.

As the world becomes smaller and increasingly interdependent, the ability to understand and communicate across ethnic, cultural, ideological, and national boundaries is an important goal of education. In addition to the exercise of learning a language, foreign language instruction also teaches students about cultural mores, which increases understanding and leads to greater communication. Therefore, a minimum level of proficiency should be sought. In general terms, this minimal level is roughly comparable to four college level courses.

An educated person in today's world should possess an understanding of and appreciation for the social diversity of this country. Diversity is one of the unique features of our country, a national treasure. Understanding the nature and value of social diversity and the closely related concepts of tolerance and equality is essential. Students need to learn the origins of social diversity, its advantages, and the ways in which all of our lives are enriched by it.

The recent increase in incidents of racism and bigotry on our college campuses is alarming and is dramatic evidence of our failure to educate our students regarding social diversity. These incidents signal the need for more aggressive action and programs that can help students understand the reasons for respecting and valuing each other's backgrounds and identities. Students will be required to complete at least one course focused on American pluralism, addressing such issues as race, gender, social class, and ethnicity.

Natural science is the study of the laws and structure of the material world. Courses in the natural sciences will provide students with information that allows them to understand the principles of physical and biological sciences, the interaction between science and technology, and the social and philosophical implications of major scientific discoveries.

In a very real and practical sense, this knowledge is essential if we are to participate fully as citizens of the world. Without this kind of information, we might be unable, for example, to understand the implications of building a nuclear power plant in our community or to choose an appropriate course of action for our own health care. Without an informed citizenry, decisions are left to the "experts" or politicians, who might have vested interests. Increasingly, educated people lack sufficient knowledge to participate fully in these types of decisions and thereby exercise their individual rights and freedoms.

A university education should include the study of the social sciences because such knowledge enhances the understanding of human behavior, the social and cultural context of that behavior, and basic social processes. The social sciences also help us understand human differences and similarities, the contemporary world, and individual and social values. Furthermore, this knowledge prepares individuals to participate in social and political communities.

Study of the arts and humanities results in an understanding that produces human imagination, activity, and culture as well as develops a humanistic perspective. Courses in this area expose students to the forms of human thought and expression, knowledge of human history, the study of different cultures, and an appreciation of the visual, spatial, musical, theatrical, and rhetorical/written arts.

As is readily apparent, the OSU model curriculum looks very different from the curriculum that currently exists in most colleges and universities: one in which students can meet their general education requirements by selecting random courses from a general list, "cafeteria style." The net effect of the current way is that students leave the university with a potpourri of general education courses that, too often, do not constitute any cohesive whole and are not structured toward any predetermined outcomes. Now let me turn to a discussion of professional education.

Professional education is an intensive experience, consisting of the mastery of a specialized body of knowledge that is both theoretical and practical (Nyre & Reilly, 1979).

Professional education includes a foundation of general education and has as a goal the preparation of competent practitioners, who possess the necessary knowledge, skill, and attitudes to function in a professional role and carry out associated activities.

In general terms, the desired outcomes of a professional education can be grouped into two areas: competencies and attitudes.

Competencies consist of the acquisition of a theoretical base and the ability to perform technical tasks, to practice with skill that is based on theory, to understand the societal context of the profession, and to anticipate and accommodate to change (Stark, Lowther & Hagerty, 1986).

The attitudinal outcomes of a professional education consist of internalized professional norms as well as the recognition of the need to increase the knowledge upon which the professional practice is based through research and internalized motivation for continued learning (Stark, Lowther, and Hagerty, 1986).

Nursing education prepares individuals to practice nursing through both general and professional education. Typically, the professional education component is built on a base of general education. However, in the recent wave of curricular reform, the prevailing thought is that general education should be part of students' education throughout their college experiences, not limited primarily to the lower division. Thus, the ideal professional education should mix professional and general education throughout the entire 4 years of study.

In 1986, the American Association of Colleges of Nursing published a document that put forth the results of a panel charged to define the essential knowledge, practice, and values for the education of the professional nurse. This document, *Essentials of College and University Education for Professional Nursing*, sets forth recommendations for both liberal and professional education in nursing.

Liberal education requirements are much like those previously mentioned and include writing, reading, and speaking English; thinking analytically; reasoning logically; understanding a second language, other cultural traditions, and oneself and others, as well as the physical world and the nature of human values; interpreting quantitative data and using computers; comprehending life and time and the meaning of spirituality; and appreciating the role of the performing arts, vis-à-vis creativity, emotional expression, and the commonality of the human experience (AACN, 1986).

Professional nursing education should provide students with opportunities to develop professional values and behaviors. The values and behaviors outlined as essential for the practice of professional nursing are altruism, equality, aesthetics, freedom, human dignity, justice, and truth (AACN, 1986). Finally, professional nursing education consists of courses that enable students to develop knowledge, clinical judgments, and skills for professional practice as they relate to patient care, both as a direct provider or coordinator of care and as a member of the profession (AACN, 1986).

Courses in the professional curriculum should be designed to provide students with the necessary learning opportunities that develop the ability to provide direct care to individuals, families, and groups who are sick or well and in a variety of settings (AACN, 1986).

As coordinators of care, professional nurses organize and facilitate care, frequently in collaboration with others. Professional courses in the curriculum should provide students with information that will enable them to do so (AACN, 1986).

Graduates of professional educational programs should aspire to improve the practice of the profession, value collegiality and work collaboratively with other health care professionals.

As a member of a profession, the professional nurse must be prepared to assume responsibility and accountability for the quality of care of patients taken on directly or given by others. The professional program should prepare nurses to apply knowledge and research findings, raise questions about care, and be familiar with the scope of their practice and the legislation that underlies that scope. Practice should reflect a knowledge of professional standards for care. Finally, nurses should be prepared to practice within the framework of professional ethics and understand the regulations applicable to themselves and to patient care (AACN, 1986).

I hope that I have made my point that appropriate outcome measures for educational programs in higher education go far beyond a licensure examination. However, I would like to make it clear that I do believe that, *if* the licensure examination accurately reflects contemporary, scientific, and state of the art nursing practice, *then* graduates of professional educational programs should be prepared to sit for the examination and enjoy a decent probability for success.

However, not all students will succeed. Indeed, in nursing we have had a much higher passing rate than many other professions, such as law, dentistry, and accounting. It is important, however, to keep in mind that the basic concept—that licensure tests for minimal competency for entry level and professional education—goes far beyond that goal.

It is not my intent to discuss the NCLEX examination at length. However, it is important, given my basic premise, that of distinguishing between licensure and professional education, to speak briefly about it. Also, it is important to understand not only the content of the exam but also the process by which test items are generated, tested, and chosen for inclusion. Such understanding is key to judging whether or not the exam reflects contemporary, desired, and scientific practice.

The NCLEX examination is based upon a definition of the nature of nursing, perceived entry-level competencies, and perceived practice requirements. In the most recent version of the NCLEX examination, the definition of nursing underlying it is the American Nurses' Association definition contained in the *Social Policy Statement.*

The declared entry-level competencies consists of the ability to identify the health needs/problems of clients throughout the life cycle in a variety of settings, to plan and initiate an appropriate action based on nursing diagnosis derived from assessment, and to evaluate the outcomes (National Council of State Boards of Nursing, 1987).

The nursing practice requirements mandate a knowledge of: nursing process, management and coordination of safe, effective care, clients' physiological and psychosocial needs, and maintenance and promotion of health.

The NCLEX test plan itself, which was derived from a task inventory job analysis of entry-level registered nurses, as identified by themselves and others (Kane et al., 1986), consists of two major components. The first is the phases of the nursing process and the second is client needs. Client needs are further broken down into safe, effective care environment, physiological integrity, psycho-social integrity, and health promotion and maintenance. The items on physiological integrity comprise almost half of the examination. If one adds to this the items on safe, effective care environment, these two areas comprise the majority of the examination.

As can be seen, the examination is much more narrowly focused than professional education. Indeed, much of the education and knowledge base of the professional nurse is never assessed, nor can it be on the examination. Yet, this knowledge is very important to quality care, the life of the individual, and society at large.

Questions can and have been raised regarding this particular emphasis as well as the process by which individual items are included or not on the examination.

Obviously, if our educational programs were primarily planned to prepare for the test, we would have much more opportunity to direct student learning into a few very specific areas. Instead, academic programs in nursing are required to reflect the requirements of the parent college or university, and to adhere to the prevailing definitions of higher education and an educated person. We would be, and to some extent have been, seriously criticized if our educational programs were exclusively technically focused and especially if they were geared only to the passing of a licensure exam.

In my discussions of licensure examinations with other academics in professional colleges, I have come to the conclusion that nursing takes performance on our licensure exam much more seriously than they do. That is not to say that other professionals are cavalier. However, they do not become alarmed when a somewhat substantial portion of their new graduates are unsuccessful on the entry-level examination. Indeed, some define that as an illustration of the rigorous standards for practice. Others more cynical define it as a way to limit the number entering the profession. Yet, they seem comfortable in the knowledge that the educational program has prepared students more broadly and believe that the preparation for the examination is the student's, rather than the program's, responsibility, and that ultimately a sound educational program will assist students to succeed. Some believe that success on the examinations may reflect some personal qualities or skills of the student, e.g., degree of preparation or test-taking skills. At any rate, they do not purport to give the same degree of responsibility for molding the professional curriculum in response to the licensing exam that nurses do. Nor would they consider using the results of such a test as a reasonable outcome measure of their educational program. Indeed, in some fields, the more prestigious programs distinguish themselves from lesser programs by labeling lesser programs as being primarily driven by the licensing exam while they dedicate themselves to theory and scientific principles.

Ultimately, nursing's future in higher education will be, in large measure, determined by our ability to adopt the norms and values of the university and to design our nursing curriculum in accordance with them. Curriculum design that adheres only to the technical requirements of a licensure exam will doom us to exclusion from the academy.

REFERENCES

American Association of Colleges of Nursing (1986). *Essentials of college and university education for professional nursing.* Washington, DC: Author.

American Nurses' Association (1979). *The study of credentialing in nursing: A new approach.* Kansas City, MO: Author.

Association of American Colleges (1985, February 13). Integrity in the college curriculum. Washington, DC: Project on redefining the meaning and purpose of baccalaureate degrees, American Association of Colleges. In *The Chronicle of Higher Education.*

Bloom, A. (1987). *The Closing of the American mind.* New York: Simon & Schuster.

Carnegie Foundation College. (1986, November 5). The undergraduate experience in America. In *The Chronicle of Higher Education.*

Kane, M., Kingsbury, C., Carlton, D., & Estes, C. (1986). *A study of nursing practice and role delineation and job analysis of entry-level performance of registered nurses.* Chicago: National Council of State Boards of Nursing, Inc.

Kelly, L. (1981). *Dimensions of professional nursing.* New York: Macmillan.

National Commission on the Role and Future of State Colleges and Universities. (1986, November 12). To secure the blessings of liberty. In *The Chronicle of Higher Education.*

National Council of State Boards of Nursing, Inc. (1987). *Test plan for the National Council Licensure Examination for Registered Nurses (NCLEX-RN).* Chicago, IL: Author.

National Endowment for the Humanities. (1984, November 28). To reclaim a legacy. Washington, DC: Study Group on the State of Learning in the Humanities in Higher Education, Author. In *The Chronicle of Higher Education, 14.*

National Institute of Education. (1984, October 24). Involvement in learning: Realizing the potential of American higher education. Washington, DC: Study Group on the Conditions of Excellence in American Higher Education, U.S. Department of Education. In *The Chronicle of Higher Education.*

Nyre, G.F., & Reilly, K.C. (1979). *Professional education in the eighties: Challenges and responses.* Washington, DC: American Association for Higher Education.

Ohio State University. (1988). *Special committee for undergraduate curriculum review: General education curriculum model.* Columbus, OH: Author.

Stark, J.S., Lowther, M.A., & Hagerty, B.M.K. (1986). *Responsive professional education: Balancing outcomes and opportunities.* ASHE-ERIC Higher Education Report No. 3. Washington, DC: Association for the Study of Higher Education.

17

SHOULD SUCCESS ON STATE BOARDS BE CONSIDERED A SIGNIFICANT OUTCOME MEASURE FOR EDUCATIONAL PROGRAMS? A REGULATORY PERSPECTIVE

Carolyn J. Yocom, PhD, RN
Director of Research Services
National Council of State Boards of Nursing
Chicago, Illinois

As a representative of the National Council of State Boards of Nursing, I will address this issue from a regulatory perspective. However, before doing so, it would be helpful to explore background information about the National Council, its purpose, its relationship to the boards of nursing, and the purpose of the licensure examinations.

The National Council is a not-for-profit voluntary organization whose membership is composed of the 61 boards of nursing in the 50 states, the District of Columbia, and four U.S. territories (Guam, Virgin Islands, Northern Mariana Islands, American Samoa). In addition, six states have two boards of nursing: one for registered nurse (RN) practice and one for practical/vocational nurse (LPN/VN) practice.

The policy-making body of the National Council is the Delegate Assembly, which is composed of two representatives from each member board. Between meetings of the Delegate Assembly, a nine-member, elected board of directors has responsibility for overseeing policy implementation and directing the activities of the organization. One example of the Delegate Assembly's responsibilities is to authorize the preparation of and to approve new or revised test plans (blueprints) that guide the content of NCLEX-RN and NCLEX-PN.

The mission of the National Council is to provide an organization through which boards of nursing can act and counsel together on matters of common interest and concern affecting the public health, safety, and welfare. This mission is put into operation through the services the National Council provides. These include: (1) the development, publication, dissemination, scoring, and provision of data pertaining to the NCLEX examinations; (2) the performance of policy analysis to identify implications of legislation or pending legislation that impacts directly or indirectly on the regulation of nursing practice; and (3) the provision of opportunities and mechanisms through which boards of nursing can share information.

One of the major ways that the National Council assists its member boards is by providing the resources and support essential for the development of a valid and reliable licensure examination—an examination that meets or exceeds accepted psychometric and legal standards for the development of licensure examinations. The NCLEX examinations aid boards of nursing to fulfill one of their major responsibilities, that of determining if candidates for licensure possess the essential knowledge, skills and abilities (KSAs) to provide minimally safe nursing care to the public at the time that they first enter practice as an RN or LPN/VN. Therefore, the sole purpose of the licensure examination is to delineate between those licensure candidates who can demonstrate minimum competence and those who cannot. Due to its psychometric characteristics, it is not appropriate to use NCLEX as an achievement test for the purpose of rank ordering candidates for licensure.

As with the preparation of all psychometric instruments, the National Council must be able to assure its membership, the public, and the nursing community of the validity and reliability of NCLEX. Support for the validity of the licensure examinations is based on a process of providing evidence that supports two essential features: (1) it measures competencies required for safe and effective performance at entry level (job relatedness) and (2) it can distinguish between candidates who do and do not possess these competencies. The second of these is addressed during item construction and evaluation and through the establishment of a criterion referenced passing standard.

However, in order to establish the job relatedness of the examination, the National Council must be able to demonstrate the linkage between examination content and the practice of newly licensed nurses. In other words, examination content must be "practice driven," not "curriculum driven." Briefly, the linkage between practice and content is supported by the chain of events identified in Table 1.

As mentioned previously, examination content must be driven by practice, not curricula. However, if curricula are in tune with practice, they should also be in tune with the test plan and therefore examination content. It is recognized that nursing education programs goals are far more reaching than preparing graduates for "the here and now" of nursing practice and the licensure examination. Nursing education programs need to provide their students with opportunities to acquire not only the knowledge, skills, and abilities that will allow them to function in the current environment but also the tools to guide nursing into the future.

Based on this background information, let us examine the powers and duties of boards of nursing with regard to setting standards in general and, more specifically, for nursing education, and relate this to the topic of this paper.

A board of nursing is mandated by state law (the nurse practice act, NPA) to protect the public's health, safety and welfare. Although the specific language of the practice acts varies from one state to another, the acts all contain language, within a section dealing with powers and duties, that state it is the board's responsibility to: (1) develop and enforce standards for nursing practice; (2) examine, license, and renew the license of duly qualified individuals; and (3) make, adopt, amend, repeal, and enforce such administrative rules, consistent with law, as it deems necessary for the proper administration and enforcement of the NPA. In addition, the practice acts in all but two states contain language that gives the board of nursing the power and duty to develop and enforce standards for nursing education. The two states not having this language are New York and Mississippi.

The nursing education standards, as established by nursing boards, serve several purposes. They include the following: (1) to ensure the safe and effective practice of nursing by graduates of nursing education programs; (2) to serve as a guide for the development of new nursing education programs; (3) to provide criteria for the evaluation of new and established nursing programs; and (4) to foster continued improvement of established nursing education programs.

While the wording of the standards vary, they commonly address such issues as qualifications of the program's administrators and the faculty, faculty-student ratios, classroom facilities, curricula, clinical practice facilities, program evaluation mechanisms, and evidence of graduates' success following program completion.

If we look at this last area, evidence of graduate success following program completion, there are a number of indicators of "graduate success" that can be used to determine if the standard has been met. These include, but are not limited to, the following: (1) results of surveys conducted to determine: (a) graduate satisfaction with their education program (i.e., did it adequately prepare them for their first position?); (b) employer satisfaction with the graduates; (2) number of graduates successful in obtaining employment; (3) number of graduates admitted to programs for advanced education; and (4) performance on NCLEX.

If you go back to the purpose of the educational standards established by a board of nursing and to the purpose of NCLEX, you will see that the use of NCLEX as one indicator of program effectiveness or quality is a valid one. The purpose of NCLEX is to determine if graduates of nursing education programs possess the essential knowledge, skills, and abilities to provide minimally safe and effective nursing care. One purpose of the education standards is to ensure the safe and effective practice of nursing by graduates of nursing education programs.

Although aggregate NCLEX results are often the most readily available indicator of program effectiveness, *they are not and should not be* the only factor taken into consideration when determining if a program of nursing education meets the established standards. However, consistent failure of a program's graduates to meet a criterion establishing the minimum percentage of graduates that must pass NCLEX may be indicative of a problem. It is for this reason that a large number of boards use aggregate NCLEX performance statistics as a stimulus for requiring a program to conduct a self-evaluation.

In a recent survey conducted by the National Council, 31 member boards indicated that their standards for nursing education include a specific criterion that educational programs must meet. Although the remaining boards do not identify a specific passing rate, their standards contain language that indicates educational programs must maintain "acceptable" passing rates and that if they don't, it could result in program review by the board.

As far as can be determined, failure to meet the NCLEX passing rate on one occasion has not resulted in withdrawal of program approval. However, a number of boards have indicated that continued failure to meet the established criterion has resulted in placing a program on probation or conditional approval status.

Clearly, graduate performance on NCLEX should not be the only criterion used to determine if a nursing education program is meeting the minimum accepted standard. However, a high failure rate may be evidence of other problems. What needs to be determined is which of the following does the failure rate represent: (1) the tip of an iceberg or (2) an ice cube that is just floating by. The only way to determine which of the two it represents is to examine the situation thoroughly.

While it is acknowledged that conducting a self-evaluation is no easy task, we know from evaluation theory that in order to determine if one piece of evidence is an indication of anything that warrants "fixing," the entire phenomenon must be examined. In the case of nursing education programs, this usually means looking at the characteristics of students (before and during matriculation in the nursing program), the curriculum, classroom and clinical teaching facilities, and faculty characteristics. Based on the outcomes of total program evaluation, then and only then should a determination be made about program quality and, if necessary, the identification of corrective measures that need to be undertaken.

So to answer the question, "Should success on NCLEX be considered a significant outcome measure for educational programs?"; the answer is "yes," but it is a qualified "yes," because it should not be used as the only measure by which program quality is judged.

TABLE 1

Process for Establishing a Link Between Entry-level Nursing Practice and Licensure Examination Content

1. Following a successful performance on NCLEX, a new graduate enters practice.

2. The National Council conducts a job analysis study using a random sample of newly licensed nurses.

3. The Examination Committee uses the job analysis study's results to examine the validity of the current NCLEX test plan.

4. If necessary, the Delegate Assembly authorizes revision of the test plan.

5. The Examination Committee prepares a draft of new test plan and disseminates it to member boards for review and input.

6. When appropriate, the Delegate Assembly approves the revised document.

7. The revised test plan is used to direct examination content.

Educational Mobility

18

AN INNOVATIVE METHOD FOR DEVELOPING A BACCALAUREATE NURSING PROGRAM AND PROVIDING PLACEMENT CREDIT FOR REGISTERED NURSE STUDENTS

P. Allen Gray, Jr., PhD, RN
Director, RN Access Program
University of North Carolina-Wilmington
Wilmington, North Carolina

People who wish to become registered nurses can participate in baccalaureate degree, associate degree, or diploma nursing education programs in the United States. In spite of this diversity in basic nursing education programs, however, there is only one registered nurse licensure examination for graduates from all programs. Having one registered nurse licensure examination ensures some similarities among the programs that prepare registered nurses, but differences do exist. Even though information is available that describes the differences in these basic nursing education programs, such differences are not clearly delineated in the minds of the general public, employers, nurses, and nursing educators (Primm, 1987).

Employers and others may not differentiate among registered nurses (RNs) who come from the three basic educational programs. Nevertheless, registered nurses from nonbaccalaureate (associate degree and diploma) nursing programs often become aware of tangible differences once they begin working. At some point in their careers, nonbaccalaureate prepared nurses generally realize that baccalaureate prepared nurses have a broader range of skills for nursing practice, have enhanced career mobility because of improved ability to compete for advanced positions, and have a foundation for graduate education in nursing. These realizations may prompt registered nurses to seek baccalaureate degrees in nursing.

Once these registered nurses return to school to obtain baccalaureate degrees, nursing educators have to determine what subject matter needs to be taught to them. It is not always possible to clearly identify what subject matter previously covered in nonbaccalaureate nursing programs exactly matches subject matter for baccalaureate nursing programs. Because of the difficulty in evaluating previous nursing education, educators in baccalaureate programs for registered nurses encounter problems in two areas: potential for redundancy in subject matter for registered nurses, and awarding credit for previous nursing education. This chapter addresses both issues.

We knew that one approach for managing redundancy used by some baccalaureate nursing programs was to negotiate agreements with nonbaccalaureate programs in their areas or regions which enabled students to move smoothly from nonbaccalaureate basic nursing programs into the baccalaureate program. Although that policy is probably helpful for a significant proportion of RN students who enroll in such a baccalaureate program, it appears to discriminate against students who come from nonbaccalaureate programs outside the baccalaureate program's region. We wanted to manage the redundancy issue in a way that would accommodate graduates from any nonbaccalaureate program including diploma schools, technical colleges, and community colleges.

Our goal was to create a baccalaureate program for RNs that: (1) would be consistent with the generic curriculum from which it was derived, (2) would minimize repeated subject matter for RN students, (3) could be completed in 1 year of full-time study after admission to the School of Nursing, and (4) would meet accreditation standards outlined by the National League for Nursing (Criteria, 1983). In pursuing our goals, we actively used curriculum design information, creativity, and intuition.

Assumptions guiding our work were that: (1) it is possible to identify knowledge RN students have already mastered, (2) it is possible to identify knowledge RN students have not yet mastered, and (3) it is possible to partition an existing generic nursing curriculum into categories of information RN students have already learned and have not yet learned. These assumptions prompted us to analyze our generic curriculum in order to produce an RN program that attained our goal of having congruent RN and generic programs.

Determining what unit of analysis to use for examining our generic baccalaureate curriculum was a most important step. We knew that faculty planning baccalaureate degree programs for RNs in schools of nursing which already have a generic baccalaureate program frequently use courses as the unit of analysis for examining their generic curriculum. Such analyses generally consist of comparing courses RNs have taken in diploma or associate degree nursing programs to courses in a school's generic baccalaureate nursing curriculum. When that approach is used, the usual outcome is to clearly show that most nonbaccalaureate nursing programs do not offer courses in leadership, research, and community nursing. Given the ease with which that conclusion can be reached, the course comparison process may seem both logical and seductively simple. Problems arise, however, in considering the remainder, and usually the bulk, of a generic baccalaureate curriculum. Courses from a nonbaccalaureate program may address many of the topics contained in generic baccalaureate courses; but baccalaureate courses often organize that information differently and present it in greater detail. For example, most nonbaccalaureate curricula emphasize sickness care for individual clients; baccalaureate programs expand the care focus to include both sickness and wellness while simultaneously expanding the client focus to include community and organizations. The course comparison process is particularly perplexing when it is used for planning a baccalaureate program for RNs because many courses in any generic baccalaureate curriculum probably contain new, as well as repetitious, information for RN students. Courses which contain a high proportion of previously learned material may frustrate RNs who expect a baccalaureate nursing curriculum to focus primarily on new information. On the other hand, if RNs are not exposed to appropriate learning experiences, they may successfully obtain the degree, but acquire a lesser knowledge base than is standard for baccalaureate nursing education. Therefore, comparing courses from previous education to generic baccalaureate courses is hardly a feasible solution to the problem of determining nursing subject matter for RN baccalaureate programs.

We declined to use courses as our unit of analysis because courses, in addition to the problems outlined above, are too general in nature to be suitable. Instead, we turned to objectives, the building blocks for curriculum. Fortunately, our generic curriculum contained clearly articulated program objectives, level objectives, and course objectives. After carefully examining each category of objective, we agreed that course objectives contained the amount of detail necessary for our purposes. We initially intended to assign each course objective in the generic curriculum to dichotomous classes of attainment by any RN student: either probably already attained or probably not attained. We soon realized, however, not all course objectives could be classified using that scheme.

Eventually, we identified three categories for classifying each of the 222 course objectives in the generic curriculum:

- objectives RNs probably had already attained
- objectives RNs probably had attained in part
- objectives RNs probably had not attained

Two faculty raters, the director of the RN program and the chairperson of the School of Nursing curriculum committee, classified the course objectives. We believed these faculty members were exceptionally well qualified to carry out the analysis because of their educational and experiential backgrounds. The director of the RN program had obtained basic nursing education in a diploma program, had graduated from a baccalaureate program for RNs, had taught in a baccalaureate program for RNs, and had worked with curriculum development and evaluation. The chairperson of the curriculum committee had taught in two associate degree nursing programs, had taught RN students in a baccalaureate nursing program, had worked closely with curriculum, and was the person primarily responsible for developing the generic curriculum which we were analyzing.

The raters independently classified each generic course objective; then, they compared category assignments for each objective. In cases of disagreement about an objective's classification, the raters discussed the meaning and intent of the objective in question and, thereby, reached consensus for every course objective's classification. Each course objective was labeled with the category to which it was assigned as well as the number of the course from which it came. Since course labels were associated with each objective, it was possible to determine what percentage of a course's objectives fell into each category.

Classifying all the course objectives in the generic curriculum completed the first step in designing our baccalaureate program for RNs. Figure 1 shows that faculty raters believed RN students would have attained approximately one-third of the generic curriculum objectives, but RNs would not have attained almost one-half the course objectives in the generic program.

Figure 2 shows that courses at the very beginning of the generic curriculum had higher percentages of their objectives classified as "probably already attained." Courses later in the curriculum had higher percentages of their objectives distributed in the "probably not attained" and "probably attained in part" categories. No courses had 100% of their objectives classified in the "probably already attained" category. Four courses (group dynamics, community nursing, research, and advanced clinical practicum) had 100% of their objectives classified in the "probably not attained" category. One course had 100%

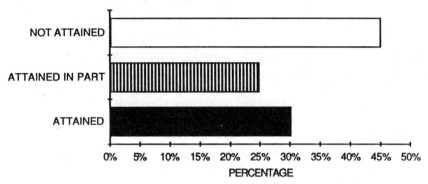

FIGURE 1
Generic Course Objective Distribution Across Classification
Categories (N=222)

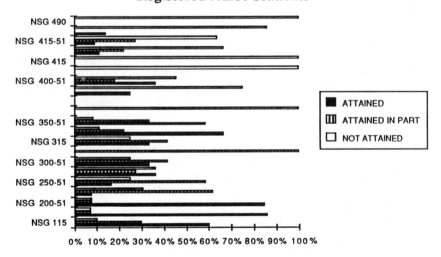

FIGURE 2
Probable Attainment Levels for Generic Course Objectives by
Registered Nurse Students

of its objectives in the "probably attained in part" category. At this point,
we agreed that courses with 70% or more of their objectives in the
already attained category would be repetitious for RN students. Conversely, courses for which RN students had attained fewer that 30% of
the objectives would contain largely new information.

   In examining course objectives, we had noted that two broad content
categories were readily apparent: nursing issues and clinical nursing.
Material dealing with nursing issues focuses on information that

enhances nursing practice; clinical nursing material focuses on direct care for clients in a variety of situations. After assigning each generic curriculum course to one of these content categories, we examined the proportions of objectives "probably already attained" for each course. Table 1 shows the outcome from sorting generic curriculum courses by content category and proportion of course objectives probably already attained. That analysis clearly revealed where strengths and weaknesses in nonbaccalaureate nursing education appeared relative to our generic curriculum.

The generic curriculum analysis now clearly indicated that one course (Introduction to Nursing) would not need to be taught for RN students. The analysis also showed that RN students would need to do coursework in areas including group dynamics, community nursing, nursing research, leadership and management, health and physical assessment, chronic illness nursing and advanced clinical practicum. We now had results similar to comparing baccalaureate and nonbaccalaureate courses; however, we believe our outcome was much more precise since it used an analysis of course objectives to determine which generic curriculum courses RN students might need.

Our next, and most challenging task, was determining what to do with the objectives from courses that had 30–70% of their objectives probably already attained by RNs. Table 1 shows five generic courses for which RN students probably had attained between 30–70% of the course objectives. Among the 85 objectives for those courses, there were 37 (43.52%) in the probably already attained category and 24 (28.40%)

TABLE 1

Distribution of Generic Courses with Objectives Already Attained by Content Categories

| Proportion of Course Objectives Probably Already Attained | Content Category | |
	Nursing Interaction/Issues	Clinical Nursing
More than 70%		Introduction to Nursing
Between 30–70%	Nursing Issues I	Clinical Nursing I
	Nursing Issues II	Clinical Nursing II
		Clinical Nursing III
Fewer than 30%	Nursing Issues II	Health and Physical
	Group Dynamics	Assessment
	Community Nursing	Chronic Illness
	Research	Nursing
	Leadership and	Advanced Clinical
	Management	Practicum

each in the probably attained in part and the probably not attained categories. Since there was no reason to work further with the 24 objectives already attained, we set them aside. We noted there were 4 objectives from the Introduction to Nursing course that were either partly attained or not attained and 9 objectives from the Nursing Process II course that were partially attained. When we added those objectives to our working pool, there were 61 objectives which RN students either probably would have attained in part or would not have attained. By associating level of probable objective attainment (partly attained or not attained) with the content categories from the previous analysis (nursing issues and clinical nursing), we created a new matrix, or framework, which allowed us to focus on information addressed by individual objectives rather than the course from which they came. Sorting objectives within the framework led us to conclude:

1. Some original, broadly stated, generic objectives could be used as RN course objectives, for example:

   Discuss health needs of families related to stage of the family life cycle.

   Source: Generic Clinical Nursing I

   Destination: RN Clinical Nursing

2. Some original, narrowly stated, generic objectives could be used as unit objectives in RN courses, for example:

   Discuss the principles of teaching-learning which the nurse must utilize in health education of clients.

   Source: Generic Nursing Issues II

   Destination: RN Transition (unit objective)

3. Some objectives which addressed the same or similar material could be collapsed or combined with each other, for example:

   ORIGINAL OBJECTIVES:

   - Perform nursing assessments of families incorporating developmental and nutritional assessment.

   - Assess communication patterns of families.

   - Incorporate family assessment into nursing of clients in acute care settings.

   - Identify examples of tertiary prevention which related to assigned clients.

   - Identify health needs of families related to stage of the family life cycle.

Sources: Generic Clinical Nursing I and III

NEW OBJECTIVE:

Perform nursing assessments of families, incorporating developmental and nutritional assessment.

Destination: RN Clinical Nursing

4. Some objectives used for RN courses needed to be stated at higher cognitive levels than those for generic courses since RNs would come to the program with considerable experiential background and would be building on previous nursing knowledge, for example:

ORIGINAL OBJECTIVE:

Formulate a Clinical Framework for Critical Care Nursing.

Source: Generic Clinical Nursing III

NEW OBJECTIVE:

Test application of a clinical framework with clients.

Destination: RN Clinical Nursing.

After considerable work, we assigned objectives to two potential courses for RN students. One course was a clinical nursing course with a lecture and a clinical component; the other was a nursing issues course. Most of the objectives for those courses were derived from course objectives originally in junior level generic courses.

This comprehensive analysis had enabled us to distill a baccalaureate nursing program for RN students from our generic nursing curriculum. The program included both courses for RN students and courses which RN students could take with generic students. Although we were quite pleased with our progress at this point, we soon realized that our product did not fit the constraints we had established at the outset of the project. Fortunately, we needed to make only one adjustment in order to keep the program length to 1 year of full-time study and to maintain a curricular sequence parallel to the generic curriculum. By moving two objectives from the group dynamics course to the RN clinical nursing course, we created a separate group dynamics course for RNs that builds on their existing knowledge of groups, carries less academic credit than the generic course, and allows us to schedule the course in a logical time sequence for RN students. This change produced two nursing issues courses for RN students: a transition course and the group dynamics course.

The transition course is similar to the one advocated by Woolley (1984) in that it establishes a curricular foundation for the remainder of the RN course sequence and is a prerequisite for all other courses RNs take in the School of Nursing. The clinical course for RNs is derived from objectives RN students probably have not attained and have partially attained from the clinical nursing courses in the first three semesters of the generic curriculum.

Table 2 shows the final course plan for our RN baccalaureate nursing program.

The innovative process described here enabled us to meet our original goals of developing a 1-academic-year baccalaureate nursing program for RN students that is parallel to and congruent with our generic curriculum. Using an analysis of course objectives from our excellent generic curriculum as the base for developing the RN program ensured a sound RN curriculum that minimized repetition of information. While we believe the process can be successfully duplicated by other schools of nursing, we cannot overemphasize the necessity for working with an existing generic baccalaureate curriculum that, in addition to having a sound curriculum plan, has clearly articulated program objectives, level objectives, and course objectives. We believe this derivative process can be a productive approach to the problem of determining what information needs to be included in baccalaureate programs for RN students. However, the process can only produce a quality outcome if it is applied to a quality generic curriculum.

Awarding academic credit for registered nurse students' previous nursing education and experience is a serious challenge. RNs returning to school to obtain baccalaureate degrees in nursing expect to receive academic credit for their associate degree or diploma nursing education. Even so, there is no standard means for identifying what subject matter addressed in nonbaccalaureate nursing programs exactly matches subject matter taught in baccalaureate nursing programs.

When evaluating baccalaureate RN programs for accreditation, the National League for Nursing (NLN) carefully examines procedures for

TABLE 2
RN Curriculum Course Plan

Nursing Issues Courses	Clinical Nursing Courses
Transition (RN)	Health and Physical Assessment
Group Dynamics (RN)	RN Clinical Nursing (RN)
Community Nursing	Chronic Illness Nursing
Research in Nursing	Advanced Clinical Practicum
Leadership and Management	

Note: RN = Course in which only RN students are enrolled.

awarding academic credit toward the degree for previous nursing education and experience. The NLN does not encourage awarding "blanket credit," i.e., granting credit merely because a student graduated from a diploma or associate degree nursing program (Resolution, 1975). On the other hand, some states, such as ours, have a Nursing Practice Act that requires baccalaureate nursing programs to award credit from previous nursing education to the baccalaureate degree in nursing (Nursing Practice Act, 1987).

As we planned our RN program, we actively explored ways to address the issue of awarding academic credit for previous nursing education. As mentioned previously, some baccalaureate programs negotiate agreements with nonbaccalaureate programs in their area so that students can move from nonbaccalaureate programs to the baccalaureate one with minimal difficulty. We wanted to maximize entrance opportunity for graduates from any nonbaccalaureate nursing program. We knew, too, that many schools use standardized tests to demonstrate that RNs have the knowledge equivalent for specific courses in a school's generic baccalaureate curriculum. That strategy works well for curricula parallel to a standardized test's organizing concepts. However, our RN baccalaureate nursing curriculum does not parallel the organizing format used for available standardized tests. We also knew it would be difficult to justify placement credit without some means for validating RN students' knowledge. After considerable deliberation, we decided to investigate using standardized tests, mainly because we believed such tests would be acceptable to accreditors and because our parent institution did not allow using locally designed tests for awarding placement credit. Our major problem was determining how to interpret results from available standardized tests for our generic nursing curriculum.

Using content analysis principles and creativity, we worked with one specific set of tests, the Nursing Mobility Profile II tests published by the NLN. The tests cover four areas: Care of the Adult Client, Care of the Client during Childbearing, Care of the Child, and Care of the Client with Mental Disorder. Two areas—Care of the Client during Childbearing and Care of the Child—are combined into one test book; the other two areas are in separate test books.

Our first task was to determine how the tests were related to our generic curriculum. By examining the content outlines published for the tests, we discovered that all the topics fell into broad content category we labeled clinical nursing courses, i.e., those which focus on direct care for clients in a variety of situations. Figure 3 shows that 60% or more of the topics from the Nursing Mobility Profile II tests were taught in the two junior semesters and the first semester of the senior year in our generic nursing curriculum. Smaller proportions of topics were in the chronic illness nursing course taught in the last semester of

FIGURE 3
NLN Mobility Profile II Topic Distribution in Clinical Nursing Courses

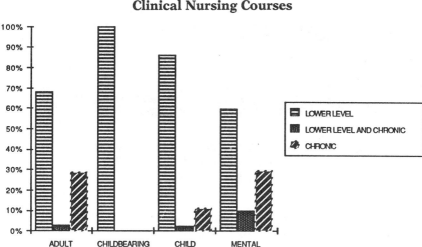

the senior year or were in the combination of lower level clinical courses and the chronic illness course.

This topic distribution analysis did not provide the detailed information we believed we needed. Therefore, we carried out a content analysis to determine how the Nursing Mobility Profile II tests reflect concepts in our generic nursing curriculum. By using a random numbers table, we identified a sample of 40% of the test items in three demonstration test books (four tests) borrowed from NLN. We then coded 233 test items using major organizing concepts from our generic curriculum's horizontal and vertical strands as classification categories. Figure 4 shows that the majority (more than 56% for any one test book) of the sample test items addressed three curricular concepts: individual, secondary prevention, and nursing process.

The content analysis outcome fit exceptionally well with the already completed course objective analysis in that both indicated RN students probably had focused in their nonbaccalaureate nursing programs on secondary prevention and probably had little or no knowledge base dealing in primary or tertiary prevention.

This evaluation of the NLN Nursing Mobility Profile II tests provided strong evidence that the tests could be used to demonstrate whether RNs admitted to our RN curriculum had a working knowledge of our generic curriculum segment, which addresses providing secondary prevention with individuals by using the nursing process. Therefore, we concluded that a passing score on the Nursing Mobility Profile II tests

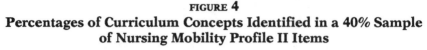

FIGURE 4
Percentages of Curriculum Concepts Identified in a 40% Sample
of Nursing Mobility Profile II Items

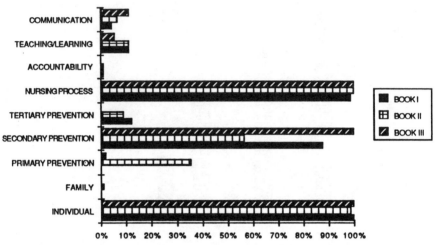

demonstrated prospective RN students had a working knowledge base for an identifiable portion of our generic baccalaureate curriculum. Because we could link the test to our generic curriculum in such a clear manner, we believed using the test would probably satisfy accreditors and would be acceptable to our university administration as a means for providing placement credit.

The next challenge was to determine a passing score on the Nursing Mobility Profile II tests . NLN, in it wisdom, provides neither a passing score nor particularly useful information for identifying a passing score with the tests. When NLN standardized the tests, it established a "decision score" which has a mean of 100 and a standard deviation of 20. Since this score is based on a normal distribution of scores, we believed it would be reasonable to consider a decision score of 80, or one standard deviation below the mean, as satisfactory performance on a given test. Since we were dealing with the entire block of tests rather than separate ones, we also decided a satisfactory composite score on the test series would consist of a decision score of 80 or above on three of the four tests. Prospective RN students who achieve a decision score below 80 on only one test are allowed to enroll in nursing courses, provided they complete remedial work in the area of weakness before placement credit is awarded. Prospective students who obtain decision scores below 80 on two or more tests in the series are not allowed to enroll in the RN baccalaureate program.

In order to satisfy the perceived NLN requirement for measuring clinical competence as well as knowledge, we devised an additional measure to determine eligibility for placement credit: the Clinical Practice Verification. The prospective RN student essentially writes a comprehensive nursing care plan for one client in a community hospital. The situation is designed so that the nurse has no prior knowledge about the client. During a period of no more than 4 hours, the nurse makes client assessments, gives medications, gathers data, and carries out routine nursing interventions. Nurses receive a set of objectives that are used both to guide the activity and to evaluate the written care plan. A minimum of two faculty members independently review the written care plans and score them either "pass" or "fail." In cases of disagreement about the final score, the faculty members either attempt to reach consensus or get the opinion of a third faculty member to resolve the disagreement.

After registered nurses have been admitted to the RN program, have satisfactorily completed the NLN Nursing Mobility Profile II tests and the Clinical Practice Verification, and have enrolled in the first course in the RN sequence, they receive 26 hours of nursing placement credit that is entered on the students' official transcripts.

ACKNOWLEDGEMENT

The author acknowledges the collaboration of Ginny Payne, RN, MSN, on the RN program development and placement credit methods described in this paper. Ms. Payne is currently Education Nurse Specialist, Pitt County Memorial Hospital, Greenville, NC. The author also acknowledges the administrative support provided for these projects by Dean Marlene M. Rosenkoetter, PhD, RN, UNCW School of Nursing.

REFERENCES

Council of Baccalaureate and Higher Degree Programs. (1975). *Resolution on the utilization of blanket credit for nurses enrolling in baccalaureate degree programs.* New York: National League for Nursing.

Council of Baccalaureate and Higher Degree Programs. (1983). *Criteria for the evaluation of baccalaureate and higher degree programs in nursing.* New York: National League for Nursing.

Nursing Practice Act. State of North Carolina General Statutes. Chapter 90, Section 1, Article 9, 90–171.19 to 90–171.47. (1987).

Primm, P. (1987). Differentiated practice for ADN- and BSN-prepared nurses. *Journal of Professional Nursing, 3*(4), 218–225.

Woolley, S. (1984). The bridge course. *Nurse Educator, 9,* 15–19.

19

PROJECT L.I.N.C. (LADDERS IN NURSING CAREERS)*: AN INNOVATIVE MODEL OF EDUCATIONAL MOBILITY

Alma Yearwood Dixon, EdD, RN**
Director of Consultation
National League for Nursing
New York, New York

The increasing demand for nursing services in hospitals and long-term care facilities, caused in part by the growing incidence of AIDS and an increasing elderly population, calls for an aggressive multifaceted effort to increase the numbers of nurses caring for patients. In New York City, this led to the creation of an innovative education and career mobility program called Project L.I.N.C. (Ladders in Nursing Careers) (Dixon & Green, 1988), which is designed to be a national and state model.

Project L.I.N.C. was initiated in the midst of the nursing shortage crisis, which has presented a challenge to nursing leaders in education and service. The urgent need to increase the supply of nurses has provided the opportunity to focus more intensely on the widely accepted concept of educational mobility. By definition, educational mobility allows an individual to climb a career ladder, with each step leading to a higher academic degree or credential and subsequent

---

*Project L.I.N.C. is a trademark of the Greater New York Hospital Association.
**Formerly, Dr. Dixon was the director of Special Studies at the Greater New York Hospital Association (GNYHA).

position. It also assumes that education is a lifelong process and implies that it may be utilized as an empowering force to enable the individual to achieve higher goals. Therefore, the concept of educational mobility is often positively linked to those individuals usually found at the bottom rungs of the ladder—e.g., the underprepared minority adult.

As early as 1972, Carnegie cited the recruitment and education of disadvantaged students as a means to help increase the number of nurses. "Equally important it would be a way of helping a group of people to fulfill their potential, as well" (Carnegie, 1972). In February 1982, the NLN Board of Directors supported the concept of educational mobility and encouraged "the preservation of this right of individuals to self-fulfillment" (NLN, 1982). Educational institutions were encouraged to provide students with the opportunity to validate prior knowledge and clinical competence. In 1988, the board reaffirmed its support of the concept and expanded its position to include the promotion of educational programs that facilitated such a movement. More recently, the Secretary's Commission on Nursing recommended a collaborative effort among state governments, nursing organizations, schools of nursing, and employers of nurses to recruit nontraditional students already engaged in the delivery of health care, e.g., nurse assistants and licensed practical nurses, and to minimize the barriers to educational mobility often faced by this category of students (Secretary's Commission on Nursing, 1988).

DESCRIPTION

Project L.I.N.C. is a collaborative effort involving over 40 hospitals and long-term care facilities that comprise the membership of The Greater New York Hospital Association (GNYHA), a metropolitan trade association representing over 100 voluntary not-for-profit institutions in New York City and surrounding communities. The institutions are linked with 20 nursing schools (LPN, associate degree, and baccalaureate degree programs) to form five consortia, one for each borough in New York City. GNYHA is the administrator and fund raiser for the entire project.

The purpose of Project L.I.N.C. is to provide educational advancement opportunities for individuals who are in entry- or midlevel jobs in nursing (e.g., nursing attendants and licensed practical nurses). This group was chosen because these individuals are currently working in the nursing field and, by definition, have made an implicit commitment to nursing. Consequently, there is a high likelihood that these individuals, once upgraded, will remain in direct patient care for a significant period of time. Also, according to hospital nursing executives in New York City, many of these individuals are known to want to upgrade.

Typically from low-income, disadvantaged backgrounds, however, they have been unable to upgrade because of financial, educational, social, or other barriers. Project L.I.N.C. was designed to eliminate these barriers.

BASIC PROGRAM GUIDELINES

Project L.I.N.C. was developed in accordance with a number of basic program guidelines agreed to by the hospitals, long-term care facilities, and schools. Many discussions centered on the needs of the employees as adult learners. The principles of adult education were stressed not only as teaching methods but also as the philosophical foundation of Project L.I.N.C. For example, it was accepted that the employees would need remedial help because of the inadequacies of their educational preparation. However, the emphasis was placed on their ability to learn, the need to identify their strengths, and the provision of resources to ensure their success. Therefore, the nine program guidelines are as follows:

1. *Counseling*: Personal support counseling services are viewed to be an essential component of this program because the employees as students may need assistance in balancing domestic, work, and scholastic responsibilities; and dealing with family matters, etc. Therefore, each of the five consortia has an educational counselor whose responsibilities include publicizing the program within institutions; selecting participants (in accordance with selection procedures agreed to by the institutions and unions); conducting diagnostic assessments; providing personal and educational counseling; assisting in school application procedures; identifying the need and making arrangements for remediation; and assisting in determining eligibility for advance placement and conducting other implementation activities.

2. *On-site instruction*: To the extent that it is feasible, courses are to be offered on-site or in locations convenient for the participants. Such courses will include those that do not require laboratories or other special facilities normally available only with a school of nursing. The intent for providing courses on-site was twofold: (1) Participants who may not have had a formal educational program for many years could begin the process in familiar surroundings, and (2) participants could have courses easily accessible to their work environments. It was understood that not all courses could or should be offered on site, especially given the benefits of interactions with other students pursuing studies in other areas.

3. *Accelerated training*: Each school is required to have a mechanism for determining proficiency and providing advanced placement in prenursing and nursing courses. The intent here is to ensure that participants will be given credit for existing skills and knowledge, and will not be required to take courses that repeat prior learning. It was recognized that two ends of a spectrum existed: Some of the participants felt that caring for patients should be validation enough of knowledge about nursing, and some nurse educators believed that nothing should be valued that a person has learned experientially or in another system. Therefore, emphasis was placed on maintaining the school's standards while utilizing existing mechanisms to determine advanced placement and award academic credit.

4. *Remediation*: Consistently, two comments were made about remediation: The nursing assistant/LPN group would probably need a lot of remedial work and, anecdotally, they would not see the relevance of remedial work to nursing.

   Although the job of the Consortium Educational Counselor was designed to be pivotal in communicating the need for remediation and facilitating the process, it was stressed that the educators played a crucial role in designing learning activities that linked basic skills to the core curriculum.

   In general, remedial courses could be provided by a school of nursing or other qualified organizations and educational institutions. Individuals requiring remediation are assisted with enrollment, registration, and other relevant processes.

5. *Special support services*: The success of Project L.I.N.C. participants depends in part on their receiving special support services, such as: (a) training in college skills, (b) orientation to the profession of nursing to enhance their understanding of the full range of professional of nursing practice (e.g., clinical judgment and decision making), (c) assistance in the transition from the participant's current role to the new role, (d) exposure to different clinical settings, and (e) educational counseling throughout the full course of study.

6. *Review courses*: Courses designed to ensure passage of the state licensing exam for nurses will be made available to Project L.I.N.C. participants.

7. *Work schedule, income, and service payback*: Lengthy discussions with nursing service and educational representatives, union officials, and others underscored the need to design a loan/service payback program that allowed individuals to work part-time and

receive a full-time salary while pursuing their studies. In light of the investment that is made in the participants, a service payback to the sponsoring institution was required.

8. *Provision of other financial resources for participants*: For most Project L.I.N.C. participants, successful completion of the program hinges in part on receiving other important resources. Therefore, resources are provided for tuition, other education-related expenses (e.g., admission fees, exam fees, lab fees, books, and supplies), and incremental personal expenses (e.g., dependent care and transportation). Under Project L.I.N.C., participants receive an expense allowance at the beginning of each semester (or other suitable arrangement) to cover these costs. The allowance will vary depending upon actual expense projections and available resources.

9. *Faculty orientation program*: Another key feature of Project L.I.N.C. is the faculty orientation program to assist faculty members from the consortium educational institutions to meet the needs of the participants in Project L.I.N.C., who are nontraditional students, e.g., students who are adults and may be minorities, underprepared, or of various ethnic backgrounds (Dixon & Green, 1988).

FUNDING

Funding Project L.I.N.C. required significant resources. GNYHA developed a broad-based funding coalition consisting of public and private sources and was awarded grants and funding commitments from the following: a private foundation, the New York State Department of Health and Labor, and a union training fund.

PLANNING

Planning began with a needs survey conducted to: (1) elicit the support of the chief executive officer and chief nurse executive; (2) determine the initial group to be targeted for beginning Project L.I.N.C.; (3) identify resources within the institutions, e.g., library facilities and computer capabilities; and (4) select the educational programs to be linked with the institutions.

Based on the results of the needs survey, the 40 institutions that decided to join Project L.I.N.C. identified the NA and LPN category as the one of greatest need. It was decided that the other rungs of the educational ladder—diploma and associate degree nurse to baccalaureate and master's preparation—would be added later. In addition, because of existing affiliations or interest in working with a specific program, the hospitals and long-term care facilities were linked with the institutions in their boroughs.

All key players were given the opportunity to comment on Project L.I.N.C. and to state their concerns, e.g., the vice presidents and directors of nursing, the deans and program directors of the educational programs, the unions, and the representatives from organized nursing. The final design of Project L.I.N.C. reflected their input.

IMPLEMENTATION

The implementation process began with the selection of the Bronx/ Upper Manhattan Consortium as a pilot. Key representatives from the hospitals, long-term care facilities, schools of nursing, unions, GNYHA, and other interested parties joined to form a Work Group to monitor the overall progress of Project L.I.N.C.

Each hospital and long-term care facility was given a specified number of slots to fill. The number allocated to each institution was determined in part by bed size. The selection criteria were developed by the hospital association, the institutions, and unions; they included the ability to be admitted to a school, seniority, satisfactory work record, and time required to complete the training program. The design of Project L.I.N.C. did not imply a structured movement from NA to LPN to associate degree to baccalaureate program. Instead, decisions were based on the applicant's interest and ability.

A brochure succinctly summarizing all of the key program elements, as well as an application, was used to begin the screening process. The brochure was carefully developed to be nonthreatening. Careful attention was paid to the words chosen, the format, and the colors used. The intent was not to be so formal as to be forbidding, or to be so casual as to appear frivolous. The brochures were distributed by each institution. While the list of candidates who were able to be admitted to a school was defined, a provision was made for employees who needed remediation prior to beginning an educational program. These employees fell into a "PreLINC" category and were referred for remedial help and can, at a later date, apply to Project L.I.N.C.

The NLN placement exam for Practical Nurse and Registered Nurse educational programs was used as an assessment tool to predict the employee's ability to be accepted into a school or be referred for remediation.

In summary, designed to be a state and national model, Project L.I.N.C. facilitates the educational mobility of health workers employed in hospitals and long-term care facilities in the New York City area who are interested in upgrading within the nursing profession. The basic program guidelines can be replicated by other institutions that seek to develop articulation programs to address the nursing shortage crisis.

REFERENCES

Carnegie, M. (1974). *Disadvantaged students in R.N. programs.* New York: National League for Nursing.

Dixon, A., & Green, B. (1988, October). Project L.I.N.C. (*Ladders In Nursing Careers*). Unpublished paper, Program Description. Greater New York Hospital Association.

National League for Nursing. (1982, February). *Position statement on educational mobility.* New York: National League for Nursing.

Secretary's Commission on Nursing. (1988, December). Final report, Vol. 1. Washington, D.C.

20

THE S-S-S CONNECTION

Celia L. Hartley, MN, RN
Director of Nursing Education
Shoreline Community College
Seattle, Washington
Margaret Stevenson, EdD, RN
Former Dean, School of Nursing
Seattle Pacific University
Julie Ann Callebert, MSN, RN
Director of Nursing
Swedish Hospital Medical Center
Seattle, Washington

As part of the program titled "Educational Systems from Uniform to Multiform" representatives of three different organizations that had worked to foster educational mobility tied with financial security for students completing an associate degree were brought together. Represented were a local community college, a private university, and a large metropolitan hospital. The following factors contributed to the success of the program:

- A collective philosophical commitment by the three organizations that these plans should (and would) come into being

- A program already in operation between Seattle Pacific University and Swedish Hospital that could be built upon

- A philosophy of education shared by the faculty at Seattle Pacific that is particularly responsive to the needs of adult learners

- Policies and practices that have been developed and implemented by Swedish Hospital that make it possible for people to attend school while working

In essence, the arrangement provides the opportunity for selected students enrolled in the associate degree nursing program at Shoreline Community College (SCC) to seek part-time employment at Swedish Hospital after completing the fourth quarter of a six-quarter program. After completing the fifth and the sixth quarter of the associate degree program, students are reimbursed for their tuition if they have continued in employment at Swedish Hospital. Following graduation from SCC, students undertake the licensing examination and continue on as Swedish Hospital employees. The following fall, the new graduates begin studies at Seattle Pacific University to complete the requirements for a baccalaureate degree in nursing, once again with financial assistance from Swedish Hospital. All organizations benefit from this relationship, but the real winners are the students. A flowchart outlining the process (Table 1), an outline of the requirements and procedures for acceptance (Table 2) and an explanation of the tuition reimbursement policy (Table 3) follow.

TABLE 1
Shoreline-SHMC-SPU Program Flowchart

	Shoreline	**SHMC**	**SPU**
Fourth quarter	N. 208-Program presented to students.	Apply to SHMC for employment as senior student nurse employee. Attend SHMC nursing orientation during break between fourth and fifth quarters. Meet with SHMC RNB Coordinator.	
Fifth quarter	Continue studies.	Work at SHMC as senior student nurse employee. Meet with SPU RNB Coordinator. Apply to School of Health Sciences. Apply to SHMC for tuition assistance.	May take nursing elective courses through SPU.

	Shoreline	SHMC	SPU
Sixth quarter	Continue studies. Graduate!	Continue employment at SHMC. Apply for tuition assistance. Apply for employment at SHMC as RN.	May take nursing elective course through SPU.
Time between Shoreline graduation and start of fall quarter at SPU.		Employment at SHMC as RN.	Take general education courses as needed to upgrade to junior status. May take nursing elective courses. Study for challenge exams. Apply for admission to SPU.

TABLE 2
Shoreline-SHMC-SPU Program: Tuition Reimbursement Policy.

Assuming active employment status at Swedish Hospital Medical Center and proof of application to Seattle Pacific University School of Nursing, Swedish Hospital will reimburse participant tuition costs:
1. To a maximum of $200 per quarter for full-time students in the fifth and sixth quarters of the Shoreline nursing program.
2. Amount to be pro-rated for part-time students, (<10 credits/quarter).
3. Reimburse student following satisfactory completion (C - Grade) of courses.

The student agrees to:
1. Work at least 1 day per week (2 days per pay period) while employed at Swedish Hospital as a senior student employee.
2. Submit grades to Swedish Hospital RN Baccalaureate Office at the completion of each quarter.
3. Commit to remaining employed at Swedish Hospital following completion of Shoreline Community College course work.

Hours Worked Per Week	*Months of Service Commitment*
40 Hours	12 Months
32 Hours	14 Months
24 Hours	17 Months
20 Hours	24 Months

4. Pay back Swedish Hospital for tuition reimbursements costs if employment is terminated before time commitment is completed.

TABLE 3
Shoreline-SHMC-SPU Program: Requirements and Procedures.

Individuals must:

1. Have attained a 3.0 grade point average in the Shoreline program.
2. Provide names of two instructors for reference purposes.
3. Meet Swedish Hospital Medical Center qualifications for employment.
4. Provide indication of past ability to concurrently work and attend school.
5. Apply to Swedish Hospital Medical Center for employment during the fourth quarter of nursing at Shoreline.
6. Apply for admission into the School of Health Sciences at Seattle Pacific University during the fifth quarter of nursing.
7. Work as a senior nursing student employee at Swedish Hospital Medical Center during fifth and sixth quarters of the Shoreline nursing program.
8. Work full-time at Swedish Hospital Medical Center after graduation from Shoreline prior to beginning the Seattle Pacific University and Swedish Hospital RN Baccalaureate Program, and a minimum of 2 days per week while enrolled in the program. Exceptions to the full-time employment requirement may be made on an individual basis.
9. Apply for admission to Seattle Pacific University by July 1st, prior to beginning the SPU Program.
10. Be accepted into the RN Baccalaureate Program no later than 6 months after beginning of employment at Swedish Hospital Medical Center.

Tuition assistance:
The 1-year length of employment requirement for the Swedish Hospital Medical Center Tuition Reimbursement Program will be waived for students participating in the Shoreline/SHMC/SPU RN Baccalaureate Program.

Themes and Images for the Future

21

NURSES IN SPACE

Martha E. Rogers, ScD, RN, FAAN
Professor Emerita, Division of Nursing
School of Education, Health, Nursing, and Arts Professions
New York University
New York, New York

In February 1957, Lee DeForest, father of modern electronics, stated:

> To place a man in a multi-stage rocket and project him into the controlling gravitational field of the moon, where the passengers can make scientific observations, perhaps land alive, and then return to earth; all that constitutes a wild dream worthy of Jules Verne. I am bold enough to say that such a man made moon voyage will never occur, regardless of all future scientific advances. (Stanton, 1989)

This was just 12 years before the Apollo moon landing.

Beware of skeptics. The world is full of famous last words.

The first studies of permanently occupied lunar bases appeared more than 20 years ago. By the 1970s, a group of experts at Johnson Space Center in Houston stated that in a few decades the term "near-earth space" will include the moon (*The planetary report*, 1988). A 1988 survey by the Public Opinion Laboratory reported that 34% of adults are interested in space exploration.

Space towns, moon villages, Martian communities are on the agenda for the 1990s. Galactic grocery stores, think tanks in space to generate creative ideas, recreational opportunities, health promotion resources—evolutionary and revolutionary—are on the way. Homo sapiens will be transcended by Homo spacialis (Robinson & White, 1986). Interplanetary and intergalactic communication with intelligent life beyond our present purview will give new meaning to citizenship in a space-encompassing world society.

New world views multiply and are directed toward complexifying wholeness. Synthesis overrides analysis. Today's innovative thinkers include such people as David Bohm, Fritz Capra, Rene Weber, Rupert Sheldrake, and Stephen Hawking. In the struggle for unity, new findings replace old facts and new interpretations emerge. Some years ago, Stephen Jay Gould noted, "Facts do not speak for themselves. They are read in the light of theory" (Gould, 1977). Changing facts are mushrooming. It seems black holes may regurgitate. Quick travel about the universe via worm holes is proposed to have practical possibilities today.

At the beginning of the present century, absolutism gave way to probability. Now probability is transcended by unpredictability (Mallove, 1989; Peterson, 1989). Cold fusion (actually proposed by Arthur Clarke, scientist and science fiction writer, some years ago) is reported and debated throughout the nation's news media.

Stan Davis (1989), looking to the future, states, "The shelf-life of an education today doesn't last a working lifetime," and emphasizes a "shift to a lifetime of learning rather than one of knowing." Maharishi International University in Fairfield, Iowa, offers experimental research outside the borders of conventional science. Education for a new reality is moving toward transcendent unity. Space is not something added to planet Earth. Rather Earth is properly integrated within infinite space. Learning within the expanding reality of space encompasses planet Earth and transcends planetary skills and knowledge. Traditional segmentation of learning is no longer adequate or even correct. The parameters of biology, physics, sociology, psychology, and the like do not lead to unity in the space world.

Complexification evolves out of nonequilibrium. It is universal and unending; continuous and infinite. Consider some manifestations of complexifying society, for example. Transition from clans and tribes to city states to nation states to planet Earth to this solar system, *ad infinitum*, provides an easy picture. Or one might examine political and governmental realities on an international basis. Are we moving toward one world? Can it be that *glasnost* has a broader significance than we have given it? Complexifying economic communities unite and merge around the planet. Increasingly, nations are joining efforts in space exploration. The new reality is infinite.

A year ago in my travels, I stayed at a Holiday Inn. In my room was the inn's worldwide directory, listing hotels, locations, features, and rates. On the cover of the directory was a picture of an astronaut on the moon. I wonder how many people have called for reservations at the Lunar Holiday Inn?

Astronauts are the precursors of spacekind: envoys of the future. How

are astronauts selected? Initially, qualifications were politically determined. Military test pilots were deemed to have "the right stuff" and to
be risk-takers *extraordinaire*. And, indeed, they were. And the Apollo
moon landing added more fuel to man's dreams.

By 1977, more flexibility in astronaut selection was appearing.
Mission specialists were introduced. These astronauts were basic scientists. Basic to selection for all astronauts was the need for team diversity.
"Composite shuttle crews are highly educated, with broad interests and
abilities beyond their specific areas of expertise" (Robinson & White,
1986). The androgynous personality is deemed most propitious, com-
bining the best of male and female stereotypes in one—more specifically, those who are goal seekers and sensitive.

A recent classified advertisement from NASA: "Wanted: pilots and
engineers preferably with military or NASA background" to become
astronauts. Of the 28 astronauts hired between 1985 and 1987, only two
(both women) came from outside NASA or the military. Nonetheless,
the need for diversity of backgrounds, precision, and teamwork were
paramount in the selection process.

At the present, there are two astronaut categories as indicated below:

1. Pilots. Qualifications for this category have changed in the past
    decade.

2. Mission specialists. People who carry out shuttle tasks. This
    category was introduced in 1977. They do not actually fly the
    orbiter, but most do have a pilot's license and many possess jet
    aircraft experience. The typical background for a mission special-
    ist includes graduate study (more master's degrees than doctor-
    ates) in engineering, math, or some science, along with several
    years of hands-on technical experience in the aerospace field.

It seems likely that there will be increased emphasis in the days ahead
for more psychological evaluations for all applicants. This takes on
considerable importance as living in space moves closer to reality.

Today's approach at NASA is oriented toward building Earthkind
habitats in space. As life evolves in space, one must then propose that
Earth-kind habitats will become outdated. Spacekind habitats loom on
the horizon. Contemporary research directed toward space dwellers of
today are concerned with such things as personal space, privacy,
human relations, isolation, the significance of color, sound, taste,
texture, and the like.

A new world view commensurate with the space age and coordinated
with the most up-to-date knowledge available must provide a substantial theoretical base for testable hypotheses in the space arena and for
spin-off to planet Earth. Planet Earth is integrated with space. This

constitutes a new synthesis. Earth is not added to space, nor is space simply superimposed on Earth. A new world view underwrites the evolutionary potential for a new species—Homo spacialis. Robinson and White propose two generations of space dwellings would be adequate. In 50 years, then, a new species may cross the horizon. Already the number of applicants for astronaut training far exceeds the available opportunities. However, opportunities for emigration to space settlements may expand rapidly once it begins. Exponential change is certainly possible and quite likely.

Where are the nurses in this scenario? In Canada, nurse representation on government space research commissions is a given. In the United States, in 1988, the First National Conference on Nursing in Space convened in Huntsville, Alabama. This conference was sponsored by the University of Alabama at Huntsville School of Nursing in cooperation with the Marshall Space Center in Huntsville. The Second National Conference is scheduled to be held April 19-21, 1990 in Huntsville. On April 18, 1989, a limited number of applicants will be able to participate in a Space Academy program designed for conference registrants.

For many years, USAF Nurses have worked at NASA as Earth-based support personnel for astronauts along with a wide range of other Earth-based personnel. These nurses have engaged in a large number of astronaut training activities. Pamela Holder's doctoral dissertation, completed in November 1988, dealt with the current role of nurses in the U.S. Space Program. Dr. Holder used an exploratory descriptive design with qualitative methodology. Common themes coming out in the findings that the space nurses in her study sample provided were as follows:

1. A support role

2. Observation/data collection responsibilities (this was largely monitoring of physical, physiological, and psychological parameters and the like)

3. Caring for the whole person (this seemed to be addictive and not holistic)

Knowledge in nursing as a science is not mentioned. Holder recommends further research and notes: "The role of ground-based nursing in the space program should be distinguished from the role of space nurse" [astronaut] (Holder, 1988, p. 10).

How should nurse astronauts be prepared if they are to be team participants in space? How, if at all, should this preparation differ from that of Earthkind nurses? It was noted earlier that Earth's inclusion in space is a process of synthesis. A space view includes spin-off to space.

Preparation of nurses for the future—both on planet Earth and in space—is a manifestation of the enlarged and new world view encompassing space. The education of all nurses—professional and technical—is properly subsumed within this new world view. The education of nurses for the space age signifies nursing as a science and an art. The science of nursing is unique in its focus of concern—irreducible, unitary human beings—Homo sapiens. (You may ask how may the predicted new species, Homo spacialis, fit?) Focus on indivisible human beings must not be confused with claims to wholes arrived at by adding parts. Wholes are clearly different from the sum of the parts. Unitary human beings are a new product. The science of nursing is an organized body of abstract knowledge. The art of nursing—the practice—is the creative use of the science of nursing for the betterment of humankind and spacekind.

Basic education for learned practice in nursing requires no less than 5 academic years with an upper division major in nursing science. Arguments over whether this preparation should lead to a baccalaureate degree or a master's degree or a professional doctorate is beside the point. Without substantive theoretical knowledge in nursing science, the particular degree is irrelevant. A laundry list of items from various sciences and tasks to be done do not constitute professional education in anything.

A broad general education foundation is essential. Knowledge of these fundamentals properly characterizes an educated person and include such goodies as literature, history, mathematics, the physical world, the social world, the psychological world, the biological world, government, religions, the fine arts, and astronomy—among a range of other subjects. The science of nursing transcends these and focuses on unitary human beings and their respective environments. The science of nursing is people-centered and community-based, whether on planet Earth or in outer space.

Learned nurses will possess a breadth of general knowledge and will be highly educated in the science of nursing. They will encompass the new world view of space. And some of these nurses may indeed be precursors of Homo spacialis. These nurses will be peer professionals of basic scientists and of learned personnel in other fields. They will be significant members of the space team, sharing equally with all other members. They will not serve as support personnel for other fields. The space teams today represent mutual respect for differences. It is the difference in knowledge and abilities that will make the learned nurse an integral part of the team and all nurses unique in the contributions to human health and welfare.

I propose that nursing's first astronauts will need a doctorate in the science of humankind/spacekind. They must be capable of filling a peer-team role. They must be able to explore the frontiers of nursing science and to be productive members in peer interdisciplinary search for new knowledge and new worlds.

For many nurses, this represents a new way of thinking about nurses and nursing. It is a contradiction of a still too widely-held attitude that includes dependency, anti-educationism, and naiveté. Euphemisms and jargon are often all too common. A new world view signifies a new reality, a new perspective. Further, with nursing as a science, a knowledge base becomes available then for nurses to be prepared to become mission specialists.

Learned nurses would be experts in the science of unitary, irreducible humankind/spacekind. The science of nursing would underwrite the practice of nurses and contribute toward determining the roles of nurses wherever people exist.

Today's nurses must ask themselves, "Will nurses be mission specialists and peer team members of the space-bound or will they be planet Earth's blue-collar support system for other fields—for astronauts who are scientists? Are nurses today in reality being trained (regardless of level of preparation) to become tomorrow's unemployables?"

Nursing: the science of irreducible human beings meets the criteria for participation as a peer-team member mission specialist. For example; nursing is unique, it is learned, it is rooted in an organized abstract system, it generates principles and theories, it leads to modalities for using space knowledge and skills to enhance the practice of nursing in space and on planet Earth.

Hands-on experience in the aerospace field, pilot experience, and the like need to be addressed. Certainly those nurses who have been and are employed at NASA have had a wide range of experiences largely as support personnel. A scientific knowledge base in nursing could make a large difference in their ability to function as peer scientists in nursing.

Scientific research is indispensable to the space effort. A new world view promises to revise both the nature and direction of research. Earthbound paradigms will not serve for this new reality.

Senator Claiborne Pell (1988) points out that "various methods are used to prevent research that is out of the mainstream from ever getting off the ground" and deplores the "gearing of all research monies toward traditional disciplines of science" (p. 6).

Florence Downs (1988), editor of *Nursing Research*, wrote "our research is replete with sophisticated methods applied to unsophisticated content" (p. 20). Research in nursing is not research in other fields. Neither is it biomedical research. Research in nursing is the study of unitary human beings and their world. Studies of what nurses do is not the study of nursing any more than studies of what biologists do is the study of biology.

Today's space research in the life sciences is more often rooted in traditional thinking. Concomitantly, new world views are forcing new definitions of science and questioning many fetishes of categorization. Altered states of consciousness are common among astronauts. Space travelers consistently return to planet Earth notably changed. Space research in the life sciences provides a means of gathering crucial in-flight data without interfering with primary mission objectives referred to as DSO (detailed supplementary objective). Reports of research in the life sciences discussed in NASA Technical Memorandum 58280 are presented under six headings, specifically: (1) Biochemistry and Phar-macology, (2) Cardiovascular Effects and Fluid Shifts, (3) Equipment Testing and Equipment Verification, (4) Microbiology, (5) Space Mo-tion Sickness, and (6) Vision ("Results of," 1987).

Space motion sickness is of considerable interest because of its frequency. Viable predictions and explanations have not yet been found. In general, the studies involve mechanistic interpretations. A re-look at this problem from a new world view with space transcendent should replace efforts to apply Earthbound criteria to space. Continu-ously complexifying wholeness opens new avenues to a future of unpredictable potentials.

The space future is here. It is fantastic and fabulous. The evolution of Earthkind to spacekind is already in process. Nor is it limited to space travelers beyond Earth. Nurses are properly an integral part of this magnificent adventure. We must envision a new future and take steps to actualize it.

REFERENCES

Davis, S. (1989, April). Envisioning the future. *Futurific*, 16–18.

Downs, F. (1988). Nursing research: State of the art. *Journal of the New York State Nurses' Association, 19*(3), 20.

Gould, S.J. (1977). This view of life. *Natural History, 52*, 20–24.

Holder, P. (1988). The role of nurses in the United States Space Program. *Doctoral Dissertations Abstract*. Huntsville, AL: The University of Alabama at Huntsville.

Mallove, E.T. (1989, May-June). The solar system in chaos. *The Planetary Report*, 12–13.

Oberg, A.R. (1989, January). Space. *OMNI*, p. 26.

Pell, C. (1988, February). First word. *OMNI*, p. 6.

Peterson, I. (1989, July). Digging into sand. *Science News, 138*, 42.

The planetary report. (1988, November/December). *3*(6), 12.

Results of the Life Sciences DSOs conducted by the space shuttle— 1981-1986. (1987, May). *NASA Technical Memorandum 58280*. NASA: Lyndon B. Johnson Space Center, Houston, TX.

Robinson, G.S., & White, H.M., Jr. (1986). *Envoys of mankind.* Washington, DC: Smithsonian Institute Press.

Stanton, F. (1989, January/February). Who believes in UFOs? *International UFO Reporter.*

22

A TRAJECTORY MODEL FOR REORGANIZING THE HEALTH CARE SYSTEM

Anselm Strauss, PhD
Emeritus Professor, Department of Social and Behavioral Sciences,
School of Nursing, University of California
San Francisco, California

Chronic illness poses a major policy issue: How can we deal with the manifestations and effects of this presently incurable and prevalent form of illness? The traditional answer is to provide efficient clinical interventions and treatments. Our health care system is based almost exclusively on this clinical orientation. Of course, a number of critics have pointed out deficiencies in the health care system concerning long-term care. The criticisms include its apparent lack of support for home health care, financial aid, and counseling for the chronically ill and their families.

My co-workers and I have joined in this chorus of criticism, arguing that the broader implications of chronic illness have not yet been fully understood. These include its implication for hospitalized care, for home care, and for an improved health care system.

I shall focus on policy issues, primarily those involving needed changes in the overall health care system—ones that nurses should be at the forefront making, both as practitioners and as political infighters. My emphasis is not on what's good for nursing as a profession as such. Rather, I am following here John F. Kennedy's famous injunction: "Ask not what your country can do for you; ask what you can do for your country"—though I will quickly add that, "What's good for your country will surely be good for you." (Or perhaps instead of saying "you"—thereby indicating that I'm not you—I should admit, after all these years, to being at least a surrogate nurse?)

I have closely studied chronic illness in hospitals and at home for some years. So I bring to this the virtues of a close-in, reality oriented eye, at least in terms of clinical and home settings. But perhaps you may sense, correctly, that this is not matched with a similar familiarity with political reality. This, however, is not meant to give an operational blueprint to policy changes; rather, it offers a vision of what is needed in the health care system. My perspective on this rests on the research my coresearchers and I have done and on its implications for health policy.

A word first concerning current criticisms about long-term care. We have looked closely at the writings of the major critics—most of them are health professionals, especially in gerontology or rehabilitation (Strauss & Corbin, 1988). Because of their training and experiences, they tend to see health policy issues largely from professionalized perspectives. So these critiques are somewhat intellectualized perspectives. Also they generally reflect an administrators' or practitioners' perspective rather than a perspective of the ill themselves.

I wish also to call attention to a paper by Bruce Vladeck (1983), "The Aging of the Population and Health Services": His position is very similar to ours though he comes at the issues from a different perspective, experience, and training. For instance, he states unequivocally that:

> Reorientation of the health care system to respond better to the problems of the chronically ill is thus one of the central challenges for medicine in the coming decades, but one that poses formidable problems, since it involves fundamental changes not only in the financing and organization of formal services, but also in the definition of roles for various groups of professional and nonprofessional personnel, the attenuation of boundaries between the medical and nonmedical spheres, and a rethinking of the balance between technical and samaritan components of medical service. . . . such programs cannot be peripheral appendages to the existing system; they must become the existing system. . . . Development of effective and affordable systems of chronic care as the core of the health care system is the central task for health policy in the coming decades. (Vladeck, 1983, pp. 142 and 148)

These critics think of failures in health care almost wholly in terms of long-term care. That is all to the good, but this tends to blur the complex relationships between acute and long-term care. It also blurs the complex relationships between the respective statuses of the ill as they pass from one phase of illness to another. The attack on the acute care perspective that dominates current health practice and policy also diverts the critics from paying much needed attention to the several phases of long-term illness, and their relationships. Indeed, there is lacking a clear and overarching conceptual framework for thinking about the total arc of work that is necessary for simultaneously managing a severe chronic illness and achieving as high a quality of life as possible.

In our latest books we have developed such a framework, around the complex concept of *illness trajectory* (Corbin & Strauss, 1988; Strauss & Corbin, 1988; Strauss, Corbin, Fagerhaugh, Glaser, Maines, Suczek & Wiener, 1984; Strauss, Fagerhaugh, Suczek & Wiener, 1985). As you may know, this concept primarily embraces the idea of a course of illness. It also includes all the work that goes into managing that course as well as the staff relationships and interactions that inevitably impact back as contingencies on both the management work and the illness course itself. This concept, and the larger framework that its elaboration represents, is firmly grounded in what living with and managing illnesses looks like to the people who suffer from severe chronic illnesses. Ill people have to think (whether constantly, frequently, or occasionally) in terms of their symptoms and disabilities as these pass through various phases and again as each phase involves a process of adjusting to the illness and making or juggling decisions in relation to it. The trajectory framework or model encompasses the entire course of illness—including all its emergent phases. It also relates the acute phases to the other phases. These phases include: prediagnostic, diagnostic, crisis, acute, comeback, stable, unstable, deteriorating, and dying.

In policy terms, this model calls for quite a radical shift of focus, organization, and resource flow in the health care system. Let me state some of more important points and implications this way:

- Chronic illness, rather than infectious or parasitic illness, is now prevalent.

- It may appear at any age, though most people experience it later in life.

- A chronic illness *persists* over a lifetime.

- When severe, it may have *many* phases: prediagnostic, diagnostic, crisis, acute, comeback, stable, unstable, deteriorating, and dying.

- Hospitals mainly care for the ill during *acute* and beginning of recovery phases, and sometimes at the very end of the dying phase.

- Periodic visits to clinics and doctors' offices are mainly for *stabilizing* the illness or slowing the patient's deterioration.

- During *all* but the acute phases, it is the ill (and families) who do the major work of managing the illness.

- It follows that the *home* should be at the very center of care. *All* other facilities and services should be oriented toward the work at home.

- In this altered division of labor, the practitioners certainly would continue to play vital and often crucial roles. So, it also follows that the *two* sides of the division of labor should be as sensibly and tightly *linked* as possible.

The last two points are of equal importance. Taken together, they imply an overall policy model that involves both care at home and care at health facilities.

Home care implies, first of all, that we view this site as *the* center of care. Second, there should be requisite provision of resources in the form of money, education, and backstopping services. Third, those resources should be in sufficient quantities and quality to enhance and augment home care management. And (a very important "and") a fourth point: these resources must be there during all phases of every long-term illness.

Home care has several components. There is the discovery, use, maintenance, and replenishing of resources in sufficient quantity and of adequate quality to get the work done in every phase of illness. There are essential work arrangements, without which the work could not get done. This illness work must be connected with other domestic work and with regard to considerations of personal identity.

Finally, and most important, all this work at home should be conceptualized as on-going. It goes on daily; it goes on forever—as long as the illness itself. For the practitioners (whether at home or at health facilities), this means their interventions must fit into and be coordinated with the on-going work of managing illness and disability in this context of daily life. Furthermore, these interventions (whether clinical or nonclinical) must be incorporated by the ill themselves into what is after all their work process.

Consider briefly what this means for the practitioners' standard term, "services," and for their much used injunction that "services should match needs." In the context of their client's overall trajectory, services as a concept can only mean that there is a division of labor in the entire work process. The ill and their intimates and caretakers do certain aspects of the work; the practitioners do other aspects. Sometimes their work overlaps. The services that the practitioner offers to, or sells to, the ill come down to resources and work arrangements that they bring to the total flow of illness work. These resources and arrangements supplement or substitute for existing ones. Matching needs with services means to provide the right resources or to institute or support arrangements that are appropriate to the on-going work flow as it streams through various phases of illness work and in relation to everyday life. Viewing services and needs in this temporal context eliminates the somewhat static and present-oriented focus that often creeps into health care and health policy.

What we are advocating is not merely building out to the home from current health facilities and agencies. It also necessitates reconstitution of the facilities and agencies in relation to much more effective and badly needed home management. This requires greatly increasing the flow of resources to the home (where right now the caretakers are preponderantly parents, spouses, and children, or in the case of people with AIDS, their lovers and families). This reconstitution of health facilities and agencies surely would entail training of practitioners to work more fully and sensitively with the ill—recognizing that the latter are true partners in working at their own care. Of course, we also need new kinds of facilities to take over—whether temporarily or permanently—when families can no longer give good care or manage their own collective lives in the face of ill members' severe deterioration or dying.

The American health care system is, in effect, mainly in the business of funding and providing acute care (that is, care during acute phases of illness). The bulk of the illness management at home concerns *other* phases of illness—which in fact constitute most of the "patient's" life. Management at home, though not as complicated as the medical management done in hospitals or clinics, is certainly as complicated in other ways. This is because of the complexity of the home context in which home management takes place, and the life-long nature of the enterprise.

Stability is the major desirable physical condition. Since specific chronic illnesses are currently unstable, we necessarily think also of the work that must be engaged in to maintain a stable condition. Much of that work is nonclinical; yet it is usually linked, in complicated ways, with the more strictly medical aspects of care. Practitioners at health facilities are skilled at managing illnesses when these are acute. They are skilled too at bringing about stability when someone is acutely ill, and adept at suggesting to the patient the best methods (regimens) for increasing the probability of the patient's maintenance of stability. Practitioners are equally skilled, for precisely the same reasons, at increasing the probability of a comeback from an acute phase as well as shortening the period of comeback before a stable level is reached. However, physicians usually, and a great many nurses still, are not formally trained in giving information or counsel to patients and kin concerning the social, psychological, and interactional aspects of chronic illness. Nor are they trained to transmit information and counsel to patients and kin that they have heard from their other patients. . . . this is exactly what happens in self-help groups and is part of the philosophy of some of those groups.

Professionals are indeed useful for slowing up and even to some extent blocking deterioration in the chronically ill. They are also helpful in increasing the probability of long periods of stability before the next drop in physical functioning. What other means then could be available to add to the health professional's armamentarium in this regard? Obviously many of the suggestions made by people who are concerned with the health of the elderly are part of the answer to that question. Yet it would pay to think of the deterioration/stability relationship not merely in terms of the elderly but also in terms of young people at different phases of illness. (If one considers the illness profiles of sufferers from severe arthritis at any age, it will be apparent that all illness phases are represented except perhaps the dying, though there may be fear of dying too. Diabetes is another instance, although typical diabetic profiles are considerably different from the arthritic ones.)

If it is true that the central drama of illness management takes place in the home, then the central actor on stage is certainly the ill person. He or she is often joined by an intimate, who not only shares the work but is indispensable to it. (If the ill are exceedingly ill, as with severe stroke or Alzheimer's disease, of course the intimate may then do almost all the work, the ill sharing little of it.) Our other research on chronic illness has taken us also into the hospital, where it has become apparent to us that the "patient" does a great deal of work. Some of it is quite visible but other work is not, although all of it is essentially unrecognized by the hospital personnel. The work is as varied as: keeping one's body absolutely still during a procedure, negotiating for pain relief, and monitoring staff's work for its competence or safety. Much of how the chronically ill patient carries out the work is based on knowledge gained from years of managing his or her illness. After leaving the hospital, of course the ill person—no longer "a patient" but a responsible person—continues with the same or altered management work. Most of the above statements can be said for the spouse or other intimates.

The point of these observations is that since the ill person is the central actor all along this life-long plot line, why not take that person's role seriously? By seriously, we mean in an organizational or programmatic sense. Today the patient's central work role is implicit or even bemoaned because of patients' frequent "irresponsibility." This is reflected in the considerable literature on so-called noncompliance. Well-intentioned but secondary efforts at teaching patients, and kin, shortly before discharge from hospital are steps in the right direction, but they hardly meet today's situation head on. Indeed the teaching there is mainly focused on the do's and dont's of the regimen. It is usually not focused specifically on the conditions that might help or hinder carrying out the regimen and controlling symptoms. Certainly it is not focused very much on how to monitor signs of clinical danger in relatively sophisticated ways.

Perhaps the most explicit recognition of the patient as an essential member of the health team is in the case of cardiac and other organ transplant patients. If one does not teach and counsel them and their spouses, and of course monitor the work they do at home, those patients will surely increase mortality statistics! Yet a recent compendium of review articles by experts on cardiac transplantation actually devoted only one slender chapter to psychosocial aspects, and the information given was by generally accepted social science standards really quite rudimentary and unsatisfactory (Evans, 1985). Even with the transplant patients, apparently the voices of patients and kin are heard *sotto voce*. Still, that situation is better than with our own interviewees, whose voices are almost wholly unheard; or if heard by practitioners and policymakers, then unnoted. The same is true, apparently, of a considerable proportion of people who have written about their own or kins' illnesses.

I touch next on a central point in what some will undoubtedly think is an impossibly idealistic set of policy suggestions. There will have to be an effective linkage of work done at home and work done in the health facilities. The problems of implementation would be, of course, enormous. This is because our health care system is not at all organized in those terms: not the facilities, not the training, not the basic perspectives of practitioners. But I believe these problems have to be faced, given the implications of chronic illness prevalence.

What is needed is for staffs in the health facilities to think in terms of clients as having chronic illness trajectories. When patients are hospitalized, they would be viewed as now in acute phases. Previously they were either in other phases (and one should discover and take them into account) or this is a first-time phase (and that will be very different from repeated acute status). Staff personnel should take seriously also the implications that they are seeing just cross sections of a trajectory that will extend far beyond the small slice of time that the patient spends at the facility. The implications of this view for care at the facilities, and for training that would fit this, are obviously far-reaching.

It is true that such change is actually coming, although slowly, since even on intensive care units the personnel are increasingly concerned with rehabilitative work in terms of patients' recovery after hospitalization. Also on pediatric cardiac units, staffs are sometimes keenly aware of the necessity of working with parents before a child is sent home with them. Alas, this is not usually characteristic of what happens on intensive care nurseries. One can also see changes in decreasing isolation of hospitals from homes in the increased development of hospital outreach programs, although these are still restricted almost wholly to immediate recovery period. Rehabilitation services are still not much oriented to the chronically ill, so this is another area where radical change needs to occur. However, rather than give a laundry list of specific suggestions, I shall only repeat that the work in health facilities and at home needs to be much more tightly interwoven. In this regard, I believe of course that innovative programs could profit from thinking in terms of the *trajectory model*.

I turn next to more traditional policy concerns. I shall make only the most general, positional statements about them, since as I've said, my aim today is only to give a basis for changing policy perspectives on chronic illness. First, the issue of funding. What is needed is a general reconsideration of—and widespread public debate about—why the overwhelming proportion of public funding goes for facilities, training, research, and practice that is so narrowly focused, in terms of all the phases of illness. There is of course the continued rising cost of health care, but this is essentially for medical or clinical care given during the more acute phases of chronic illness. Nobody yet knows whether shifting of funds toward home care would stop or slow down the inflation of costs, but at least the money might be more effectively spent. When cost-cutting policies such as those that have dominated recent governmental regulations are considered in the future, focused questions might well be asked about what the effect of new measures will be on the recovery and stability of patients discharged from disproportionately costly hospital care. We should also ask whether the new measure might not actually add to the costs of containing illness.

My coresearchers and I agree with long-term care critics of the health care system that there should be a redirection of funding toward home care and toward the improvement of nursing homes, especially by staffing them with genuinely trained and psychologically sensitive nursing personnel. Not only should actual services be funded but surely appropriate financial mechanisms could be instituted for giving exhausted spouses and caretakers periods of respite. These mechanisms should also keep the greatly deteriorated ill out of nursing homes by minimal financial support of them or their families. Financial support is also needed for training the health workers who visit homes, so that they will understand better how to give appropriate home care.

Another prominent issue debated in the health arena is that of equity, or equal opportunity for access to health care services. Advocacy of equity is deeply rooted in a humanitarian reform tradition that goes back many decades. Much as I also subscribe to the demand for equity, I do believe its proponents are much too focused on access to acute care. They will say, perhaps, "first things first." Our answer to this argument is that demands for equity should be updated to include equitable and appropriate care for all phases of life-long illness. Even if complete justice were to prevail for accessibility to health facilities, this would hardly solve the health problems of poorer Americans. Even the working class ill who do have fair access to facilities and coverage for medical expenses need much more by way of diverse services and supportive arrangements. The impoverished certainly have more chronic illnesses, are sicker from them, die earlier from them, and quite obviously need more than acute care services. The same can be said for a multiplicity of American ethnic groups. Each of these has different cultural traditions that sometimes affect the services they need and how they should be offered. For such cultural reasons, some minority groups find the health services less accessible than they should be. This is part of the equity problem too. The traditional views of equity, in short, need some rethinking.

The same is true of another issue, that of bioethics. Mainly the debate that has arisen around medicine in relation to questions of morality has been focused on medical high technology and its impact on dying. If we think in terms of chronic illness, ethical considerations are really associated with each of its several types of phases. For instance, should the ill be told about all the potential side effects of cancer therapy? Or only some? When? How? By whom?

Apropos of medical technology, the unceasing debate over technological assessment is confined essentially to the cost and safety issues of technology devoted to acute care. Thinking in terms of chronic illness would enlarge greatly the sphere of action for people who are in other phases of illness—much as in recent years, the disabled have profited from relatively simple but wonderfully effective new inventions like walkers and electrified wheelchairs. Only now are we beginning to get devices or tests that allow self-monitoring at home of blood pressure or of diabetic signs. There should be concerted attempts to develop and improve such low-cost technologies for home use, and funding for the necessary research and training of the ill.

In closing I will note an assumption that lies behind my central argument. For infectious and parasitic disease, the aim of medicine is to save people or, in less extreme illnesses, to get them well more quickly. For chronic illness, however, the clinical aim must necessarily be something else. Even if survival or delaying death is the immediate aim, nevertheless once the patient is out of danger, clinical effort can only slow up deterioration, mitigate symptoms, or relieve symptoms. This means an improved quality of life because of fewer restrictions on what the body can do, and thus what activities can be engaged in, accomplished, or enjoyed. Improving the quality of life is what the health practitioners are really in the business of doing—as are the ill and their assisting families. This, too, is what the health policy makers should strive to contribute toward. An undue medical-clinical focus (and a rather narrow focus on acute illness at that) is both a betrayal of what modern medicine is capable of contributing to and a betrayal of public trust in the health professions. [Indeed, this is the import of the title and contents of our old book, *Chronic Illness and the Quality of Life* (1984).]

I realize, of course, how difficult it is to make any major change in the nation's approach to illness, considering the financial and other problems that it faces, plus the diverse political stances, plus the length of time it takes for any large-scale change to occur. Right now seems the most hopeless of times for advocating such views—for at this point, families are being brutally forced by the cutbacks in hospitals and agencies to shoulder increasingly the burdens of their own care. Nevertheless, it is our hope that if enough people say the same thing for a long enough time, those with the power to make a difference will hear the message and begin to institute the necessary reforms. The inexorable impact of an aging population should certainly hasten that day.

To be chronically ill in America is not just to be an individual struggling against fate; it is a societal condition shared by all the chronically ill. No industrial country seems to have solved the psychological and social problems attending and affecting their physical plight, by instituting and maintaining even approximately effective and humane organizational arrangements. This country certainly has not done so. One of our national dilemmas rests on the propensities to further extol and even glorify individualism, on the one hand. There is, on the other hand, a seeming reluctance to yield to collective action and governmental implementation, while really pursuing these forces with vigor and receiving their benefits willingly. These contradictions have entered into the nation's handling of the chronically ill. Characteristically our technologically and organizationally oriented society has better confronted chronic illness itself than the associated issues that concern the chronically ill. We let the ill more or less fend for themselves, for they are presumably responsible individuals and citizens. This literally forces them to be the centrally responsible agents in their own care—rather than admitting that they are the central workers whose efforts are abetted by the health practitioners. This policy strategy fails to face up to the far-reaching implications of chronic illness prevalence. It avoids our more fully meeting the responsibilities of a genuinely humane society, does it not?

REFERENCES

Corbin, J., & Strauss, A. (1988). *Unending work and care: Managing chronic illness at home*. San Francisco, CA: Jossey-Bass.

Evans, R. et al. (Eds.). (1985). *The national heart transplant study: A final report*. Seattle: Battelle Human Affairs Research Center.

Strauss, A., & Corbin, J. (1988). *Shaping a new health care system.* San Francisco, CA: Jossey-Bass.

Strauss, A., Corbin, C., Fagerhaugh, S., Glaser, B., Maines, D., Suczek, B., & Wiener, C. (1984). *Chronic illness and the quality of life.* St. Louis, MO: Mosby. Revised edition.

Strauss, A., Fagerhaugh, S., Suczek, B., & Wiener, C. (1985). *The social organization of medical work.* Chicago: University of Chicago.

Vladeck, B. (1983). The aging of the population and health services. *Annals, 468,* 138-48.

23

HEALTH POLICY ISSUES TOWARD THE YEAR 2000

**Brigadier General Clara L. Adams-Ender,
MMAS, MSN, RN**
Chief, Army Nurse Corps
Falls Church, Virginia

It was both humbling and an honor to present the Dorothy J. Novello lecture on health policy issues at the 1989 National League for Nursing Convention. This paper is an adaptation of that lecture.

Some of you who are "vintage people," as I am, may remember Dr. Dorothy Jean Novello. I would like to summarize some highlights of Dr. Novello's outstanding nursing career after graduating from St. Joseph's Hospital School of Nursing in Pittsburgh. She went on to earn baccalaureate and master's degrees at Duquesne University and a doctorate degree from Harvard. Her nursing experiences were many and quite diverse in both nursing service and nursing education. The sustaining highlights, however, were in nursing education where she was an instructor, assistant professor, lecturer, teaching fellow, and professor. She subsequently became dean of the Erie Institute for Nursing, Villa Maria College, Erie, PA. Dr. Novello's productive nursing career reflects a person who has always been willing to give more than she received in ensuring quality health care to clients. She was once chairman of the Pennsylvania State Board of Nurse Examiners; First Vice President, Health Systems, Inc. of Northwestern Pennsylvania; consultant to the Western Interstate Council on Higher Education; and member of the Board of Trustees of the Commission on Graduates of Foreign Schools of Nursing. She was active in community planning for health care delivery in Pennsylvania and served on numerous committees and commissions for mayors, governors, and health care organizations. Dr. Novello was a past president of the National League for Nursing, a noted author and expert in health care policy issues. She was a visionary and could always be counted upon to present the "big picture" so that approaches to resolving challenges in health care would be comprehensive. Her untimely death a few years ago left a tremendous void in health policy leadership. We must all become aware of these issues and be willing to give the time and effort necessary to gain successful outcomes for which Dr. Novello gave so much of her time and effort.

The crisis in health and the many disturbing and often conflicting trends in health care are well known to us. I would like to discuss some of those trends and health policy issues today in an effort to increase your awareness of some major challenges that must be faced in health care in the year 2000.

Just before I begin the serious side of this lecture, I would like to share some significant information about other changes that have been witnessed by a group that I will call the survivors! This piece is dedicated to all those born before 1945. It was taken from the *Tri-County News* and it is entitled for "All Those Born Before 1945: We Are the Survivors!!" Consider the changes we have witnessed: We were born before television, before penicillin, before polio shots, frozen foods, Xerox, plastic, contact lenses, frisbees and the pill! We were born before radar, credit cards, split atoms, laser beams and ball point pens; before pantyhose, dishwashers, clothes dryers, electric blankets, air conditioners, drip-dry clothes and before man walked on the moon. We got married first and then lived together. How quaint can you be? In our time, closets were for clothes, not for "coming out of." Bunnies were small rabbits and rabbits were not Volkswagens. Designer jeans were scheming girls named Jean or Jeanne and having a meaningful relationship meant getting along well with our cousins. We were before house husbands, gay rights, computer dating, dual careers, and computer marriages. We were before day-care centers, group therapy, and nursing homes. We never heard of FM radio, tape decks, electric typewriters, artificial hearts, word processors, yogurt, and guys wearing earrings. For us, time sharing meant togetherness—not computers or condominiums; a chip meant a piece of wood!! In 1940, "Made in Japan" meant junk and the term "making out" referred to how you did on your exam. Pizzas, McDonalds and instant coffee were unheard of. We hit the scene when there were 5- and 10-cent stores, where you bought things for five or ten cents. For one nickel, you could ride a street car, make a phone call, buy a Pepsi or enough stamps to mail one letter and two postcards. You could buy a Chevy coupe for $600, but who could afford one? A pity, too, because gas was 11 cents a gallon. In our day, cigarette smoking was fashionable, grass was mowed, coke was a cold drink, and pot was something you cooked in. Rock music was a grandma's lullaby and

AIDS were helpers in the principal's office. We were certainly one before the difference between the sexes was discovered, but we were surely before the sex change; we made do with what we had. And we were the last generation that was so dumb as to think you needed a husband to have a baby. No wonder we are so confused and there is such a generation gap today!! But we survived!!! What better reason to celebrate?

That bit of levity will serve as a launching point for this chapter on health policy issues toward the year 2000. Although written with much wit and humor, there is also the wisdom that underscores the stark realities of how our society, our world, our morals and values have been altered in varying degrees over the years. If some of you are like me and were born before 1945, you are probably lamenting about those days and are asking yourselves, "Whatever did I do to inherit the world in such a state?"

I want to familiarize you with significant health care policy trends and issues and to discuss specific actions which must be taken to demonstrate sound leadership and resolution of challenges in the 21st century. In order to accomplish these objectives, however, some background information and an update on the issues in the health care industry must be provided.

There were two significant reports that were published in the past year that I want to share with you. I would also urge you to read them in depth, both for further information and for a thorough knowledge of the issues in health care today. The first report is from the deliberations of a group called the National Leadership Commission on Health Care. The group consisted of concerned citizens who first met together in 1986 to address three major problems of health care: cost, quality, and access. The group members were a distinguished group of leaders from many disciplines—health care providers, business, law, economics, politics, ethics, and labor. (I also thought it significant that there were no nurse members on this commission.) The commission, during its deliberations, agreed on a vision of a healthy society in the 21st century, one that promotes preventive care and healthy lifestyles through vigorous public education and that operates an innovative and efficient health care system which provides universal access to a basic level of appropriate and affordable care.

They concluded that the main problems in health care today were problems of cost, access, and quality. They explored these factors in depth. There has been a dramatic increase in health care expenditures, far above general inflation rates over the past few years. The causes of these cost increase include general inflation, accelerated inflation in medical care prices, aging of the population, patient demand, increasing physician supply, the use of inappropriate care, the practice of defensive medicine, and advances in medical science leading to expensive new technologies. In 1988, Americans spent $550 billion on health care (11.4% of the GNP), far more than any other country in the world. If trends continue, health care costs will double in 1995 and triple by the turn of the century, reaching $1.5 trillion in the year 2000 (15% of the GNP and $5551 spent on each American). One must also underscore the fact that costs of health care have escalated without a significant and measurable improvement in the health of the nation. Cost containment has become the rallying cry as a result. The prospective pricing system based upon diagnostic-related groups has been put into place. Tight controls on budgets for hospitals and on new construction have been activated. Other mechanisms include health maintenance organizations and increased managed care, decreased inpatient census and an increase in outpatient visits.

A second disturbing element is access to care. There are growing numbers of Americans without health insurance. It is estimated that 37 million Americans (one-third of them children) have no health insurance and perhaps an equal number of Americans are underinsured. This means that one out of every four Americans may be either uninsured or seriously underinsured. Consequently, they do not seek health care until they are quite sick, which leads to an increased burden on the health care system.

The quality of health care was the third area of concern. There is insufficient information on the quality and outcomes of medical services and insufficient means of monitoring the quality of care and fostering its improvement. Increasing reports and stories of unnecessary or equivocal care have led to the need to overhaul the rudimentary quality control system. Hospitals have traditionally focused only on how care was delivered. They have only just begun to measure the impact of that care on patient outcomes. Patients also have few tools to help themselves assess the quality and appropriateness of their treatment.

The commission concluded that the critical problems of cost, access, and quality of health care in American today present a clear and compelling case for change. These interrelated problems cry out for interrelated solutions. Piecemeal approaches will no longer suffice.

The commission rendered its report in January 1989. It marked the first time in 35 years that payers and providers of health care worked together to produce a plan for a new health care system for the country. The recommendations rendered by the commission were presented as a proposal. The strategy contained some critical and interrelated elements:

- Provide universal access through a new universal access (UNAC) program to a basic level of health care regardless of income.

- Spread the cost of paying for such universal access by requiring all employers and all Americans above 150% of the poverty level to pay a fee to finance health care of those not covered by insurance.

- Provide financial incentives to encourage employers to extend coverage to all employees.

- Use state agencies to implement the proposal.

- Establish a multifaceted cost containment strategy.

- Improve quality by greatly increasing research on effectiveness, appropriateness, and quality of care and publicizing results.

- Use existing private organizations and public agencies to support research and development of national guidelines on the appropriateness of health care.

- Control costs by spreading information into the marketplace.

- Encourage the widespread adoption of promising state-level reforms of malpractice laws.

The second significant report on health care rendered recently was from the Health and Human Services Secretary's Commission on Nursing. In January 1988, President Reagan asked Health and Human Services Secretary Otis Bowen to bring together a commission to determine the state of nursing in America and to report back to him and the Congress by the year's end. The report is significant because it was the first nursing report mandated from a federal agency headed by a cabinet member. The commission was directed by Dr. Carolyne Davis and consisted of distinguished health care providers, consumers, and federal employees. It was also the first time that the military nursing services were represented in a major nursing study—the Chief Nurse of the Air Force was appointed as a commissioner to represent the military nursing services.

The commission deliberated, held hearings, took testimony, analyzed data, and rendered a final report in December 1988. I urge you to read the report in full; however, there is an excellent summary of the major findings in the January 1989 issue of *Nursing Health Care* ("Not Just," 1989). The major findings of the commission about the state of nursing were:

- There is a shortage of nurses in America.

- The shortage of nurses is the result of the rapidly increasing caring needs of an aging population, new technologies and treatment possibilities, and the emergence of new diseases, especially AIDS.

- The shortage of nurses is apt to worsen before it gets better.

A summary of the major recommendations follows:

1. *Appropriate utilization of nursing resources:*
   - Use RNs for the purpose for which they were educated—to provide professional nursing care.
   - Provide adequate support services, including automation and labor-saving devices.
   - Use appropriate mix of nursing personnel.
   - Seek other measures to increase the productivity of registered nurses.

2. *Improve nurse compensation:*
   - Compensation is currently inadequate—both salaries and benefits.
   - Of increasing concern is severe wage compression over the span of a nurse's career. An example of salary compression is most evident in a survey conducted by the Wyatt Company in July 1988 that found the average starting salary for staff registered nurses (RNs) to be $22,300, the average salary was $26,000, and the average maximum salary was $30,000. In essence, while most other professionals can expect at least to double their starting salary during a career, staff RNs can expect an increase of only $8000 during a career!
   - The commission noted that the occurrence of nurses leaving their careers due to compensation levels happens more often than in other professions.

3. *Improve health care financing:*
   - Support compensation, especially in nursing homes and health care sectors.
   - Improve and increase funding for nursing education.

4. *Nurse decisionmaking:*
   - The commission commented that the failure to recognize the need for nursing input on the part of health care delivery organizations, physicians, and health care policymaking bodies has contributed to problems in recruiting and retaining nurses, hindered their development and care orientation and limited the efficiency and effectiveness of patient care delivery.
   - Nurses can make unique, critical, and effective contributions to the health care system—until now they have been virtually an untapped resource for the policymaking arena.

5. *Development and maintenance of nursing resources:*

   - Federal government effort is needed to spearhead a sustained effort to monitor the nurse labor market, collect data, and conduct research on demand as well as supply in nursing practice.

   - There should also be follow-through on implementation of the recommendations of the report of the commission.

The final statement of the commission's report is emphatic: "It is the sincere belief of the commission that the health of this nation will be at risk if the changes suggested in these recommendations do not occur." The statement speaks directly to the importance of nursing to the health care system. In essence, as Barbara Jordan stated when she keynoted the ANA Convention last year, "Nursing is the linchpin of the health care system. Without nursing, there would be no health care system."

There are significant issues and trends that must be addressed in health policy formulation today. I will address some that are technological, educational, and labor and work related. As technological trends are viewed, computers will be commonplace, smaller, and more widely used in health care delivery. New production technologies will continue to be adopted. Computer-aided design in industry will shorten the amount of time between an idea and finished design. All of the technological knowledge we work with today will represent only 1% of the knowledge that will be available in 2050. There will be greater emphasis upon specialization in health care because of a knowledge explosion. Automation technology is not the wave of the future—it is the wave of the present. One must ask oneself: In my work environment today, can I operate more than the telephone?

Educational trends predict that there will be expanding education and training throughout our society because of a rapidly changing job market. Education costs will continue to rise and there will be increasing pressure to control costs. Two-year colleges and associate degrees will grow. Loans rather than grants will constitute the main source of student financial aid. There will be educational reforms as a result of the information economy's call for skilled workers. More students will be actively recruited to science and engineering schools. There will be a severe shortage of qualified teachers, and estimations of 1,000,000 new teachers are cited as being needed between 1989 and 1993. Educational institutions will be more concerned with ways to assess outcomes and effectiveness of educational programs than ever before.

Labor force and work trends are as revolutionary as technological and education trends. There will be increased specialization within professions, especially in health care, legal, and engineering fields. In nursing, for example, the body of knowledge to be mastered to excel precludes excellence across all areas and the needs of patients will dictate it. Arguments about entry levels into nursing practice will be overcome by events. This will be good for nursing because a rise in educational level will raise the status of nursing as challenging and meaningful work and ultimately lead to increases in salaries and benefits.

There will be a steady growth of the service sector. The Bureau of Labor Statistics shows steady growth to 88% of the labor force by 2000, with approximately 1,000,000 new jobs being created in the less skilled and laborer categories. In addition, there will be an increased use of assistants. The growth of health care professionals is most dramatic. The need for registered nurses alone is expected to be over 650,000 by the year 2000. Other categories of health care workers expected to increase significantly are physical therapists, X-ray technologists, pharmacists, occupational therapists, medical technologists, and other laboratory personnel.

The rise of minorities and women in the labor force will be dramatic. It is estimated that women will constitute 64% of the work force by the year 2000. It will still be important for nursing leaders to do whatever is necessary to attract, recruit and retain women and minorities in the health care professions.

Specific actions need to be taken in order to demonstrate sound leadership in health care in the 21st century. The director of the specific actions must address the issues most dramatically affecting health care today—cost, access, and quality. The specific actions must also demonstrate knowledge of societal trends and issues which impact health care as well as a vision of a future for a healthy society.

Waterman in his book, *The Renewal Factor*, proposes some overall actions for any organization or business to flourish and grow. I would like to share them with you because they seem most appropriate for resolving the challenges of the health care industry by inviting us to foster a renewed environment in our work settings. Waterman states that the first action in fostering renewal within an organization is to promote teamwork. Teamwork is the key to progress in organizations. Studies have shown an inverse relationship between a low amount of teamwork and a high amount of turf-battling, jealousy and in-fighting in organizations. Companies and organizations with good teamwork and cooperation (starting at the top) enjoy a terrific multiplier effect; a close-knit group accomplishes far more than a throng of divided and disjointed staff members. Lack of teamwork in health care results in poor outcomes, especially for patients. Those organizations or groups that promote teamwork enjoy communication which seems uncanny to outsiders; important ideas move like quicksilver; and shared experiences and team-building are promoted. Leaders who promote teamwork do not operate under the strain of fear and anxiety that they will be replaced or rivaled in their jobs. They know that they need not be superhuman and that they must use the talents and abilities of the capable people with whom they have surrounded themselves. Promotion of teamwork at all levels of leadership is essential in the renewal of the health care business. We do not stand taller by putting others down.

A second action that Waterman states is essential in renewing organizations is the development of trust relations. All "we/they" barriers must be removed because they are detrimental to change and renewal and because they fragment an organization. Leaders must use all of the work force to determine the most feasible course of action. The strength of actions is participation across all organizational boundaries. When trust relationships get off track or are nonexistent, meaningful communication ceases and drastic steps must be taken to return the organization to a high level of productivity. Leaders who develop trust relationships also empower their work forces by allowing them to act on their own behalf after they have been given appropriate direction. These leaders may then sit back and manage the results.

Waterman's third essential action for renewing organizations is to be involved in politics. Involvement in politics is necessary at all levels, whether we like it or not. Politics is really the effective use of information (usually about people, relationships, and situations) to accomplish goals and objectives. There are some mixed reviews on the necessity of politics in organizations. Some executives insist that they are essential, others want to eliminate politics as much as possible. One certain fact is that politics is always present in organizations. Renewal organizations tend to make politics a positive factor by emphasizing and promoting teamwork. Political behavior in organizations is perfectly natural and legitimate and is sometimes the only way to get things done. Nurses must learn to have greater respect for political power in organizations at all levels and to use politics to accomplish their goals and objectives. It will be increasingly necessary to do this to be successful leaders in health care in the 21st century.

Waterman's fourth and final essential action for renewal of organizations is to pursue and wield power. If I were now to check the galvanic skin responses of most nurses after saying the word "power," they would probably be off the scale for many. We seem to desire to be powerless leaders, a concept that is doomed to failure. My definition of power is the ability to affect outcomes. Nurses desire and seek the ability to affect outcomes. Consequently, nurses must seek and wield power. Pursuit of power is a necessity in our delivery of nursing care and patient advocacy roles. The ability to seize and wield power must be evident in the day-to-day pursuit of collective goals. Power must also be shared. It was Lord Acton who said, "Power tends to corrupt and absolute power corrupts absolutely." The last thing that the health care system needs right now for renewal is nurses who are unwilling to share power, who are insecure and unwilling to speak out on the tough issues, and who are unwilling to negotiate. Our importance in the health care system has been acknowledged and firmly established. We must continue to demonstrate responsibility and accountability by doing whatever is needed to provide the necessary input into policy decisionmaking. Pursuing and wielding power is one of those necessary actions. Active involvement in the pursuit of power improves with experience. One must also learn to celebrate successes in this regard and to reward oneself for having performed well.

In summary, the major issues of health care toward the year 2000 are cost, access, and quality. The significant trends in society with a direct impact upon health care are technological changes, changes in education, and alterations in the labor work force. For the health care industry to experience renewal and reform, leaders must promote teamwork, develop trust relationships among all its workers, be involved in politics at all levels, and pursue and wield power. We face some tough and challenging days ahead as leaders in health care. However, no one is better able to meet those challenges than we are (or they would be here doing it instead of us!). Consequently, we must continue to demonstrate the caring, concern, and commitment necessary to tackle the tough issues daily—and win!!

REFERENCES

Not just another nursing report. (1989). *Nursing & Health Care, 10*(1), 11–12.

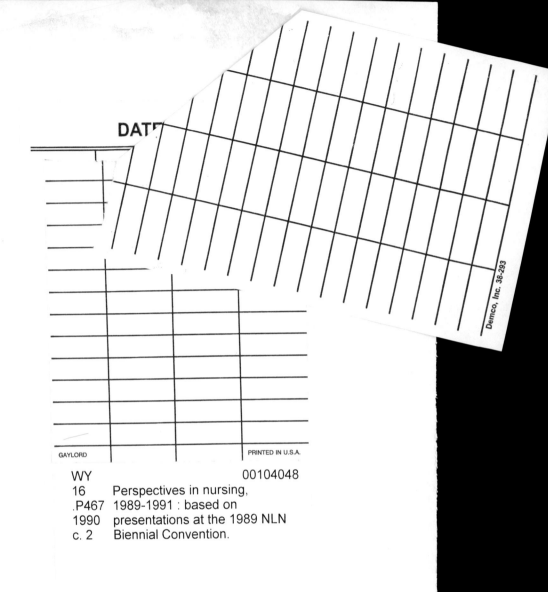